L'anglais à l'IFSI

Guide pratique à l'usage des Instituts de Formation en Soins Infirmiers

Didier CARNET
Agrégé de l'Université, Maître de Conférence

Jean-Pierre CHARPY
Agrégé de l'Université, Maître de Conférence

Anaïs CARNET
Enseignante à la Faculté de Médecine de Dijon

Philip BASTABLE
Enseignant à la Faculté de Médecine de Dijon

Faculté de Médecine de Dijon
Université de Bourgogne

ellipses

Remerciements

Les auteurs tiennent à remercier vivement les collaborateurs francophones et anglophones qui par leur relecture minutieuse et leurs suggestions précieuses leur ont permis de nombreuses mises au point durant la rédaction de ce livre :
Françoise DURIEZ (Cadre Supérieur de Santé, IFSI Dijon), Marilyn THWAITES (RGN).

Ils tiennent à remercier tout particulièrement :
Martine GOISET pour ses compétences informatiques,
Louise PIANETTI-VOARICK pour ses illustrations.

ISBN 978-2-7298-66549

32, rue Bargue 75740 Paris cedex 15

www.editions-ellipses.fr

Préface

Parmi les éléments importants de l'arrêté du 31 juillet 2009 relatif au diplôme d'état d'infirmier, figure la création d'un module d'anglais destiné à être enseigné tout au long des trois années d'études dans les Instituts de Formation en Soins Infirmiers. La justification de ce module (6.2) tient à la nécessité d'une part d'optimiser les capacités des futur(e)s infirmier(e)s à pouvoir communiquer avec des patients dont le français n'est pas suffisant, d'autre part de donner les bases suffisantes pour lire et comprendre des articles et des documents professionnels en langue anglaise.

L'anglais est aujourd'hui dans tous les domaines la langue universelle. Son apprentissage durant le cycle secondaire donne aux bacheliers une base scolaire qu'il faut ensuite conforter par un enseignement plus orienté vers le langage professionnel. Cet ouvrage propose, grâce à un équilibre pertinent entre l'apprentissage du vocabulaire médical si spécifique, la mise en situation clinique, l'abord des techniques en soins infirmiers, la lecture de documents professionnels (protocole, articles) et des exercices judicieusement choisis, une formation progressive couvrant l'ensemble du programme d'anglais des trois années d'étude.

Les auteurs, Didier Carnet et Jean-Pierre Charpy, Maîtres de Conférence à l'Université de Bourgogne et Anaïs Carnet et Philip Bastable, enseignants à la Faculté de Médecine de Dijon sont chargés d'organiser et de dispenser l'enseignement de l'anglais médical avec une spécificité locale : cet enseignement y est continu tout au long du cursus de six années des deux premiers cycles. Ils ont donc acquis une expérience pédagogique et docimologique sans équivalent pour transmettre aux étudiants les bases théoriques et pratiques de la langue anglaise à usage professionnel. Ils sont auteurs de nombreux ouvrages, articles et documents pédagogiques très utilisés par les collègues médecins. Ils exploitent tous les outils disponibles, en particulier audio, vidéo et numériques, pour enrichir leurs documents et faciliter un apprentissage dont on ne peut concevoir qu'il soit exclusivement livresque.

L'étudiant en soins infirmiers trouvera dans ce remarquable manuel l'ensemble des bases nécessaires à la communication dans son cadre professionnel. Il pourra exploiter les ressources pédagogiques les plus modernes lors de son travail personnel afin d'améliorer sa syntaxe ou sa prononciation.

Les français ont la détestable réputation d'être particulièrement réfractaires à l'apprentissage des langues étrangères. Gageons que grâce à ce nouveau document pédagogique particulièrement réussi, les étudiants en soins infirmiers sauront faire taire les plus pessimistes et surprendre les enseignants.

Professeur Frédéric HUET, Doyen

Faculté de Médecine. Dijon

Université de Bourgogne

Table des matières

Avant-Propos

Le présent ouvrage est divisé en trois parties destinées à couvrir les trois années des études à l'IFSI. Ce manuel est destiné à l'enseignement de l'anglais (Unité d'Enseignement 6.2) dans le cadre de l'universitarisation de la formation en soins infirmiers (arrêté du 31 juillet 2009, voir programme officiel ci-après).
Les enseignants d'anglais intervenant dans les IFSI ou dans la formation continue des infirmiers / infirmières y trouveront une banque de données correspondant aux activités habituelles des soins infirmiers.
Cet ouvrage peut également être utilisé par l'infirmier / infirmière en exercice désirant perfectionner son anglais en travaillant en auto-formation. En effet, ce manuel donne accès à un grand nombre de situations authentiques diversifiées par le biais de dialogues, de documents vidéo accessibles en ligne (en utilisant le lien indiqué) et de brochures professionnelles. Les termes les plus usités et les plus utiles sont traduits à la suite de chaque document, et repris systématiquement dans l'index en fin de manuel.
La pratique systématique des compétences linguistiques telles que définies par le cadre européen commun de référence (listening, reading, spoken interaction, spoken production, writing) devrait permettre aux étudiants ayant certaines lacunes d'atteindre les niveaux B1-B2 de ce cadre de référence à l'issue de la première année.
Les documents que nous avons retenus sont progressivement plus complexes afin de contribuer à l'enrichissement médical et linguistique des étudiants et de leur permettre d'atteindre le niveau C1 en fin de cursus.
Dans les 15 premiers chapitres (S1-S2), tous les thèmes abordés (les études d'infirmier, les différents services de l'hôpital, l'évaluation de la douleur, les instruments médicaux, les systèmes corporels...) sont présentés par le biais d'un dialogue et d'un document vidéo accessible en ligne. Des exercices écrits et un travail oral en binôme sont systématiquement proposés pour faciliter l'acquisition du lexique spécialisé mobilisé et des structures utiles présentées.

Ces chapitres fonctionnent de la manière suivante :

- L'axe central de chaque chapitre repose sur un dialogue : « Nursing in action » et une vidéo portant sur un même thème spécialisé. Ces thèmes correspondent aux programmes de la première année des études en soins infirmiers, car les auteurs sont convaincus que les connaissances et compétences linguistiques ne doivent pas être dissociées des connaissances et savoir-faire infirmiers.
- Deux « boîtes à outils » accompagnent systématiquement ces textes. Elles fournissent :
  - un élargissement du vocabulaire spécialisé thématique : « Build your vocabulary » ;
  - une aide à la communication par le biais d'un précis fonctionnel : « How to... ? ».
- Le vocabulaire spécialisé et/ou usuel est systématiquement traduit en français : « Word list » et repris en fin de manuel sous forme de glossaire. Les principales formes irrégulières des verbes et quelques collocations utiles sont disponibles en fin de manuel.
- Quelques exercices à dominante lexicale ou fonctionnelle permettent de s'assurer systématiquement de l'acquisition des étudiants.
  L'ultime exercice : « Do it yourself », s'appuie sur un travail en binôme et permet le réinvestissement des notions lexicales et fonctionnelles étudiées dans le chapitre par le biais de travaux d'interaction orale. Cet exercice communicationnel encourage la prise de parole autonome des étudiants.

Les huit chapitres suivants (S3-S4) sont davantage orientés vers les techniques professionnelles et s'appuient sur les connaissances que les étudiants auront acquises progressivement au cours de leur première année d'étude.
Chaque chapitre comprend :

- Des explications et démonstrations de diverses techniques de soins infirmiers : « Nursing skills », (injections, pose de cathéter, pansements, prise de sang, administration de médicaments...) sont abordées par le biais de documents visuels professionnels.
- Une vidéo authentique traite du même thème.
- Le vocabulaire spécialisé et/ou usuel est systématiquement traduit en français : « Word list » et repris en fin de manuel sous forme de

glossaire. Un élargissement lexical est également proposé sous la rubrique « Additional vocabulary ».

- Des exercices de traduction spécialisée d'articles professionnels (écrite et/ou orale) permettent de s'assurer de l'acquisition lexicale et des connaissances liées à la pratique professionnelle des étudiants.

  Un dernier exercice : « Pairwork » entraine les étudiants à communiquer sur leur pratique professionnelle à partir des documents visuels proposés au début du chapitre.

Les sept derniers chapitres (S5-S6) sont directement focalisés sur le métier d'infirmier / infirmière et présentent les différents rôles auxquels seront confrontés les futur(e)s IDE.

Chacun de ces chapitres comprend :

- Un document authentique (brochure, notice explicative, posologie...) permettant aux étudiants de consolider leurs connaissances lexicales et professionnelles : « Document for nurses ».
- Une vidéo portant sur un aspect du métier d'infirmier / infirmière.
- Le vocabulaire spécialisé et/ou usuel est systématiquement traduit en français : « Word list » et repris en fin de manuel sous forme de glossaire. Un élargissement lexical est également proposé sous la rubrique « Additional vocabulary ».
- Des exercices de traduction spécialisée (écrite et/ou orale) d'abstracts permettent de s'assurer de l'acquisition lexicale et des connaissances liées à la pratique professionnelle des étudiants, et leur faciliteront la traduction en anglais de l'abstract du mémoire de fin d'étude visant à l'obtention du grade de licence.

  Un dernier exercice, « Pairwork », met en scène de façon communicationnelle des situations réalistes auxquelles les futur(e)s IDE seront confronté(e)s.

Les étudiants en soins infirmiers peuvent redouter d'avoir à faire face à des documents variés et parfois ardus en anglais. Les auteurs espèrent que, grâce au travail diversifié et progressif proposé dans ce manuel, les étudiants et étudiantes en soins infirmiers seront en mesure de passer de l'apprentissage de l'anglais à l'IFSI à une pratique concrète en anglais dans le contexte des soins infirmiers. Ainsi, ils/elles seront armés pour accueillir tout patient parlant anglais et faire face à toute situation pour laquelle l'anglais peut se révéler nécessaire.

Textes et programmes officiels
(arrêté du 31 juillet 2009)

6. Méthodes de travail et Anglais

6.1 Méthodes de travail : 25 heures
6.2 Anglais : 60 heures

Unité d'enseignement 6.2

Semestre : 1 à 6
TD : 60 heures
ECTS : 10

Objectifs

- Communiquer en anglais dans le domaine de la santé et des soins
- Etudier et utiliser des articles professionnels en anglais
- Eléments de contenu
- Vocabulaire professionnel courant dans le domaine de la santé et des soins
- Expression anglaise dans le domaine de la santé et des soins
- Lecture et traduction d'articles professionnels
- Lecture de documents (fiches, procédures, ...)
- Recommandations pédagogiques

Cette UE vise à donner à l'étudiant des bases d'anglais dans le domaine de la santé et des soins.

Modalités d'évaluation

S1 : présence et participation active
S2 : présence et participation active
S3 : épreuve de connaissance du vocabulaire professionnel courant
S4 : traduction écrite ou orale en français d'un article professionnel
S5 : présentation en anglais d'un article professionnel
S6 : rédaction de l'abstract du travail de fin d'étude

Première année

S1-S2

Chapter 1

THE STUDENT NURSE / L'ÉTUDIANT INFIRMIER (ÈRE)

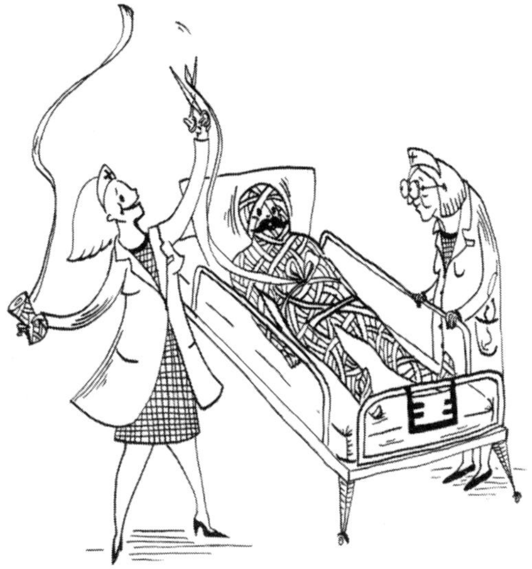

BUILD YOUR VOCABULARY

nursing	soins infirmiers
practical nursing skills	techniques infirmières
nursing school / school of nursing	Institut de Formation en Soins Infirmiers (IFSI)
nurse	infirmière
male nurse	infirmier
student nurse (GB) / nursing student (US)	étudiant infirmier / infirmière
qualified nurse	infirmière diplômée
State Registered Nurse (SRN) / Registered General Nurse (RGN)	Infirmière Diplômée d'Etat (IDE)
Licensed Practical Nurse (LPN)	infirmière auxiliaire (Canada)
nurse's aide (GB) / auxiliary nurse (US)	aide soignante
staff nurse	infirmière hospitalière
sister /senior nurse (GB) / head nurse (US)	infirmière en chef
nursing officer	cadre de santé
district nurse / community nurse (GB) / visiting nurse (US)	infirmière à domicile / infirmière libérale
theatre nurse (GB) / scrub nurse (US)	instrumentiste / panseuse
circulating nurse	infirmière de bloc

NURSING IN ACTION

In the amphitheatre, at the nursing school...
Good morning everyone. Welcome to the nursing school.
You've all made the wonderful decision to study nursing. It's a very noble but **demanding** profession and I'm sure you'll all have **rewarding** careers.
There are **countless** opportunities for qualified nurses, not only in this country, but all over the world – the USA, Australia, South Africa.
During your studies, you will learn the basics of nursing, but later on, once you've obtained your diploma and become an SRN, a State Registered Nurse, you can specialize in a **wide range of fields**.
Let me give you an **overview** of the programme.
During your first year, you'll be studying biology and medicine as well as practical nursing **skills**.
In addition to the theory, every **semester** you'll have a five-week **training period** in one of the **departments** of the hospital to get some practical experience. These training periods are very important and each will be **assessed** and will thus contribute to your final **mark** for the year.
Your professional skills are of course essential, but your interpersonal skills will also be **taken into account**.
You are the person the patients have most contact with, so you need to show understanding, to be reassuring, to be a **caring** person.
For those who show management skills, there are possibilities for career advancement. You can go on to become a sister in charge of a whole **ward**, and why not a senior nursing officer with more responsibility and mainly administrative and teaching **duties**... and there are plenty of opportunities to work in the private sector too. Do you have any questions?
OK, no questions for the moment. So, I wish you all success in your studies and in your professional careers. My door is always open if you need to speak to me about anything at all.

Word list

demanding	exigeant
rewarding	gratifiant, enrichissant
countless	innombrable
a wide range of fields	un large éventail de domaines
overview	vue d'ensemble
skills	compétences
semester	semestre
training period	stage
department	service
(to) assess	évaluer
mark	note
(to) take into account	prendre en compte
caring	attentionné
ward	unité de soins
duties	tâches

VIDEO

Truth about being a nurse

http://www.youtube.com/watch?v=NoHCOwdHk8o

Script:
For a Licensed Practical Nurse, or LPN, helping people is the top priority. **Overall**, LPNs provide physical and emotional **care** for **the sick**, **injured** and handicapped.
Specific duties **range from** taking a patient's **blood pressure** to starting intravenous fluids, to assisting **emergency room staff** during operations.
Because a patient's **well-being** depends greatly on quality care from LPNs, responsibility and emotional **strength** are pre-requisites for the job.
If you are interested in this career, you must be observant, able to **notice** changes in a patient's condition, and take quick and decisive action in any situation.
Since LPNs play an active role in teaching people how to stay **healthy**, you should also be willing to **be called upon** to teach family members basic nursing tasks or to speak to children about good health and **diet habits**.
This occupation is not without its risks, as you must be prepared to work with people with infectious **diseases**. However, by following **safety** policies and procedures, an LPN's job can be kept both **safe** and satisfying.

Word list

overall	globalement / dans l'ensemble
care	les soins
the sick	les malades
the injured	les blessés
(to) range from... to	varier de... à / aller de... à
blood pressure	tension artérielle
emergency room	les urgences
staff	le personnel
well-being	bien-être
strength	force
(to) notice	remarquer
since	puisque
healthy	en bonne santé
(to) be willing to	être prêt à
(to) be called upon	être sollicité
diet habits	habitudes alimentaires
disease	maladie
safety	sécurité
safe	sûr / sans danger

HOW TO ... ASK QUESTIONS?

1. **Yes/No questions** > **Auxiliary + subject + verb**

Ex.:

Do you smoke?
Are you taking any medications?
Could you take off your shirt, please?
Have you ever had an operation?

2. **Wh/How questions** > **Question word + auxiliary + subject + verb**

Ex.:

How did you break your leg?
Where does it hurt?

Watch out: if the question word is the subject, the basic structure changes
> **Question word + verb**

Ex.:

What is your name?
Who is your family doctor?

EXERCISES

1. Find the correct question.

1. Yes, it's a very demanding job.
2. She's been working as a circulating nurse for five years.
3. Her name's Marilyn Thwaites.
4. No, they haven't been assessed yet.
5. Yes, she can (give injections).

2. Translate the following questions.

1. Aimerais-tu être infirmière hospitalière ou infirmière à domicile ?
2. Dans quelle unité de soins travaille l'instrumentiste ?
3. Comment s'appelle l'infirmière en chef ?
4. Dans quel service as-tu fait ton stage ?
5. Quelle note as-tu eu à ton stage ?

DO IT YOURSELF

Pair work: Student 1 missed the welcome talk; he/she asks **student 2** a few questions about what was said.

Ex. *Will we have any training sessions?*

Chapter 2

A GUIDED TOUR OF THE TEACHING HOSPITAL / VISITE GUIDÉE DU CHU

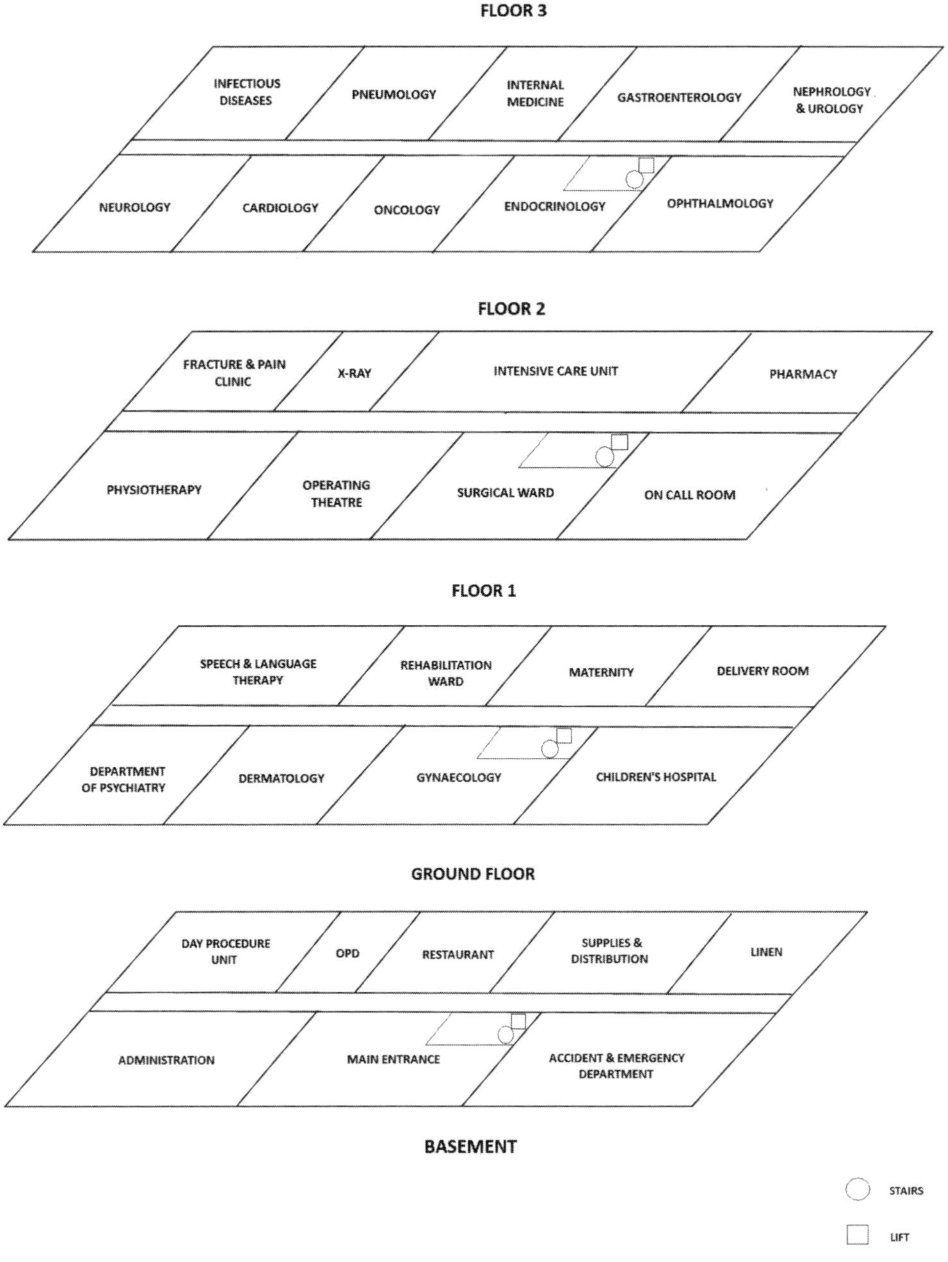

BUILD YOUR VOCABULARY

floor / storey (US)	étage
ground floor (GB) / first storey (US)	rez-de-chaussée
first floor (GB)/ second storey (US)	premier étage
basement	sous-sol
lift (GB) / elevator (US)	ascenseur
stairs	escalier
corridor	couloir
on the left	à gauche
on the right	à droite
turn left	tourner à gauche
turn right	tourner à droite
go straight ahead / on	continuer tout droit
near / close to / next to	près de
over there	là bas
in front of	devant
opposite	en face de
on the other side of / across from	de l'autre côté de
behind	derrière
between	entre
at the far end of	au fond de

NURSING IN ACTION

Reception Hall - a senior nursing officer is giving a group of first-year student nurses a guided tour of the teaching hospital...

Right, here on the ground floor you will find the administration offices.

The lifts to the other floors, including the basement are just over there on the right, and the stairs just opposite the lifts.

This corridor **leads to** the Accident and Emergency department, so those who have a training period there, just go along to the end of the corridor and **introduce yourselves** to the head nurse, Joan Bakewell.

The children's hospital is on the first floor, so those **assigned to** this department, go up to the first floor, turn right when you get out of the lift and **knock on** the second door on your right. This is the **nursing station**. Nurse Alice Greenway will explain your duties to you.

For the others, your training period is in the dermatology department. Go up to the 1st floor and follow the signs. You'll meet Brian Salcombe, who will be your tutor.

For lunch, there is a **staff canteen,** next to the restaurant on the ground floor. There are **microwave ovens** and fridges if you want to bring a **packed lunch**, or if you like you can buy a **meal** for £2.75.

So have a good day.

Word list

(to) lead to	mener à / conduire à
(to) introduce oneself	se présenter
(to) assign to	affecter à
(to) knock on	frapper à
nursing station	poste de soins infirmiers
staff canteen	cantine / cafétéria du personnel
microwave oven	four à micro-ondes
packed lunch	panier-repas
meal	repas

VIDEO

Auckland city hospital tour

http://www.youtube.com/watch?v=RUL0hs5rz_8

Script:
Welcome to National Women's at Auckland City Hospital. The **purpose** of this DVD is to show you where to park your car when you're coming in labour and how to get up to **Labour and Birthing Suite**. Auckland City Hospital is located on Park Road Grafton. Park your car at **gate 1** main entrance. You may want to leave a prewritten note for security. Let security know that you are here. Labour and Birthing Suite and Women's **Assessment** Unit are on level 9. If necessary, push the **override button** which takes the lift straight to the ninth floor. Turn right into Labour and Birthing Suite. After 8 pm, the doors are closed, press 1 on the **keypad** to contact staff. When admitted, staff will welcome you to the unit. **Support person** has then to return to the car and move it to carpark A. Support person returns into the hospital from the back entrance. If the door is **locked**, press 1 for exit. Follow the blue **broken line** to the level 1 lift and return to level 9.
Rooms and services:
There are 14 Labour and Birthing rooms, 6 of these have a **pool**, all have a **shower** and toilet. Let your **lead maternity carer** know if you plan to use the pool. Birthing aids are available. Music and aromatherapy are OK to bring. Mobile phones are OK to use.

Word list

purpose	but / objectif
in labour	en travail
Labour and Birthing Suite	salle de travail et d'accouchement
gate 1	porte 1
assessment	évaluation
override button	bouton d'accès direct
keypad	clavier
support person	accompagnant
locked	fermé à clef
broken line	ligne discontinue
pool	baignoire
shower	douche
lead maternity carer	responsable des soins

HOW TO... ASK QUESTIONS?

1. **Yes/No questions in the simple present and simple past > Auxiliary do / does / did + subject + verb**

Ex.:

Do you smoke?
Does the surgeon operate on Saturdays?
Did you take your medication today?

2. **Wh/How questions > Question word + auxiliary + subject + verb**

Ex.:

Where does it hurt?
How did you break your leg?

Watch out: if the question word is the subject, the basic structure changes
> **Question word + verb**

Ex.:

Who lives here?
What killed her?

EXERCISES

1. Answer the following questions using the indication in French.

Ex: Where's the lift?
(juste derrière vous)
It's right behind you.

1. Where's the ophthalmology department?
(de l'autre bout du couloir)
2. Where's the ENT department?
(au premier étage)
3. Where's the waiting room?
(à droite en entrant)
4. Where's the cafeteria?
(en face de l'administration)
5. Where's the neurology department?
(en haut des escaliers, à gauche)
6. Where's the head nurse?
(certainement au poste de soins infirmiers)
7. Where's the X-ray department?
(au sous-sol)

2. Find the correct question.

1. I have three children, 2 boys and a girl.
2. I take aspirin every day.
3. She works at the hospital.
4. The pain started last Saturday.
5. Nurse Brown worked here from 2006 to 2010.

DO IT YOURSELF

Pair work 1: Use the plan of the hospital and ask the receptionist how to reach specific parts of the hospital.

Ex. Student 1 (visitor): Excuse me, could you tell me the way to the delivery room, please?
Student 2 (receptionist): Take the lift to the first floor. Turn right when you come out of the lift and the second door on the left leads to the delivery room.

Pair work 2: Student 1 describes a route without giving the destination. Student 2 listens to the instructions and gives the destination.

Ex. Student 1: Go through the main entrance door and take the lift to the second floor. Get out of the lift, turn left and walk straight on to the end of the corridor. Take the last door on your right.
Student 2: I'm in the fracture and pain clinic!

Chapter 3

HOSPITAL ADMISSION / ENTRÉE A L'HÔPITAL

BUILD YOUR VOCABULARY

admissions desk	bureau des entrées
admission form	formulaire d'entrée
triage nurse	infirmière au triage
family doctor / general practitioner (GP)	médecin généraliste
referring doctor	médecin référent
personal details / particulars	renseignements personnels
surname / family name / last name (US)	nom de famille
given name / first name (US)	prénom
gender	sexe
male	masculin
female	féminin
country of origin	pays d'origine
date of birth (DOB)	date de naissance
marital status	situation familiale
maiden name	nom de jeune fille
married	marié(e)
single	célibataire
divorced	divorcé(e)
widowed	veuf / veuve
occupation	profession
home address	adresse personnelle
professional address	adresse professionnelle
relative	parent
next of kin	parent le plus proche
contact person	personne à prévenir
relationship with the patient	lien de parenté avec le patient
admission reason	raison de l'hospitalisation
national health insurance number	numéro de sécurité sociale
private health insurance	assurance complémentaire / mutuelle

NURSING IN ACTION

Accident and Emergency Unit…
Mrs James: Could you look at my son, please – he pulled a **pan** of **boiling** water onto himself. We put **plenty of** cold water on it, but we didn't **dare** to **undress** him.
Triage nurse: Right, let me see – he's **scalded himself pretty badly**, there are **blisters** on his **scalp**, his face and his **neck**.

Are you Mr James?
Mr James: That's right
Nurse Gregory: Could you go to the admissions desk and give your particulars to the secretary so that we can open a **medical file** for your son.
Mr James: Of course.

At the admissions desk
Mr James: Hello, I've just brought in my son and the triage nurse asked me to come to you to fill in an admission form.
Secretary: Hello, could I have your son's full name and address, please?
Mr James: Certainly! Henry James, and the address is 63 Richmond street, Lancaster.
Secretary: What's his date of birth?
Mr James: He was born on the 15th of May 2007.
Secretary: Is there a phone number where I can **reach** you during the day?
Mr James: Yes, my **cell phone** number is 07912 386 455.
Secretary: Should I put you or Mrs James as the next of kin?
Mr James: Put my wife's name, Susan James. You can contact her at 01772 122 377.
Secretary: Who's your family doctor?
Mr James: Dr Stevenson, 10 High Street, Lancaster.
Secretary: What happened to your son?
Mr James: He scalded himself.
Secretary: Has he been hospitalized before?
Mr James: No, he's never had any problems so far.
Secretary: So, he's not taking any **medication**?
Mr James: No, nothing.
Secretary: Are his vaccinations **up to date**?
Mr James: I'm not sure. I'll have to check with my wife.
Secretary: And does he have any allergies that you know of?
Mr James: No, I don't think so.
Secretary: Do you have private medical insurance?
Mr James: Yes, We are with Bupa.
Secretary: Thank you, Mr James, that's all for the moment.

Word list

pan	casserole
boiling	bouillant
plenty of	beaucoup de
(to) dare	oser
(to) undress	déshabiller
(to) scald oneself	s'ébouillanter
pretty badly	assez sévèrement
blisters	cloques / phlyctènes
scalp	cuir chevelu
neck	cou
medical file	dossier médical
(to) reach	joindre
cell phone	téléphone portable
medication	médicaments / traitement
up to date	à jour
Bupa= British United Provident Association	mutuelle britannique

VIDEO

Hospital Admission

http://www.youtube.com/watch?v=PnJRebZGje8

Script:
When you're admitted to the hospital you'll be **assigned** a room and a bed number and be taken there by **wheelchair**. A nurse will welcome you to the unit and begin your nursing assessment. She'll take your **vital signs**, ask you about your **medical history**, do a physical examination; they may very well start an **intravenous line**, an **IV**, just so that doctors will have quick access if your medical situation **requires** that. The nurse or an aide will help orient you to the room, show you where the **call button** is to **summon** help, how to operate the television and generally get you comfortable in bed. If you're allowed to walk around, you'll be shown where the **restroom** is, and you may even be **advised** by the nurses as to when to expect your doctor to first visit you.

Word list

wheelchair	fauteuil roulant
vital signs	signes vitaux / constantes
intravenous line (IV)	intraveineuse / perfusion (perf.)
(to) require	nécessiter / exiger
call button	sonnette
(to) summon help	appeler à l'aide
restroom (US)	toilettes / WC
(to) advise	informer / conseiller

HOW TO... EXPRESS NUMBERS?

1. **Cardinals from one to 99**

one	eleven		
two	twelve	twenty	twenty-one
three	thir**teen**	thirty	thirty-two
four	f**our**teen	f**or**ty	forty-three
five	**fif**teen	**fif**ty	fifty-four
six	sixteen	sixty	sixty-five
seven	seventeen	seventy	seventy-six
eight	eighteen	eighty	eighty-seven
nine	nineteen	ninety	ninety-eight
ten			

Hundred, thousand, million, billion, trillion... are invariable (no **s**) when they are preceded by a number.

Ex. Two **hundred** patients
They are used in the plural when they are followed by **of + noun**.
Ex. **Hundreds** of patients

A **comma** can be used to separate large numbers into hundreds, thousands, millions...
Ex. 3,246,502 = three million, two hundred and forty-six thousand, five hundred and two.

In English, decimals are expressed with **the decimal point** (and not with a comma, as in French). In spoken English, you must say **point** and pronounce each digit separately.
Ex. Serum biochemistry showed increased troponin I at **1.78** μg/L with normal creatinine and electrolytes. (= **one point seven eight** micrograms per litre)

2. **Ordinals** are used to express position in a series, dates and the majority of fractions..

1**st**	first	11th	eleventh	21**st**	twenty-**first**
2**nd**	second	12th	twel**f**th	22**nd**	twenty-**second**
3**rd**	third	13th	thirteenth	23**rd**	twenty-**third**
4**th**	fourth	14th	fourteenth	24th	twenty-fourth
5th	fi**f**th	15th	fifteenth	25th	twenty-fifth
6th	sixth	16th	sixteenth	30th	thirtieth
7th	seventh	17th	seventeenth	50th	fiftieth
8th	eighth	18th	eighteenth	100th	hundredth
9th	ninth	19th	nineteenth	1000th	thousandth
10th	tenth	20th	twent**ie**th	...	...

In number-only dates, there is a major difference between British and American English. People say:
Ex. **12.10.2009** = the twelfth of October two thousand and nine (GB)
12/10/2009 = December ten two thousand and nine (US)

Telephone numbers are given one digit at a time in groups of 3.
In British English, 0 is pronounced like the letter O (oh).
Ex. 07912 386 455 = oh seven, nine one two, three eight six, four double five

EXERCISES

1. Write these numbers in words

1. 3,698
2. 15/12/2007
3. 06/22/2010
4. 3.1416
5. 3/5
6. 18,130
7. €2,000
8. 01772 234 543

2. Fill in the blanks with words seen above.

1. To make a good cup of tea, the water has to be ___________.
2. After the long walk, I had ___________ on my feet.
3. I'm afraid my vaccinations are not ___________.
4. Your _____________ is incomplete, I need your DOB.
5. I need the address of your next of ___________.
6. My husband died a few years ago, so I am ___________.
7. I tried to phone several times, but I couldn't __________ Dr Jones.

DO IT YOURSELF

Pair work 1: Number dictation: **Student 1** writes eight numbers like the ones above, and dictates them to **student 2** without showing them. Once you've finished, check that you've written the right numbers.

Pair work 2: Student 1 is the patient; **student 2** is the admission secretary. Ask questions and give answers to fill in the following admission form.

<table>
<tr><td colspan="2">DEPARTMENT : ________________________________</td></tr>
<tr><td>SURNAME : ________________________

GIVEN NAME : _____________________

DOB: _____ / ______ / ______
AGE :____

HEALTH INSURANCE NUMBER :
____
GP : ____________________________</td><td>MARITAL
STATUS ________________

OCCUPATION :
____

HOME ADDRESS :
____
—
____
—

PHONE NUMBER :
__________________</td></tr>
<tr><td colspan="2">NEXT OF KIN :
____

CONTACT PERSON : Mr / Mrs / Ms
____

RELATIONSHIP WITH PATIENT :
______________________________</td></tr>
<tr><td colspan="2">Admission date: _____ / ______ / ______

Admission reason:
____
____</td></tr>
</table>

Chapter 4

THE HUMAN BODY / LE CORPS HUMAIN

BUILD YOUR VOCABULARY

Put the following words in the picture below:
abdomen / ankle / arm / calf / chest / elbow / finger / foot / forearm / hand / head / heel / hip / knee / leg / lower limb / neck / shoulder / thigh / thumb / toe / upper limb / waist / wrist

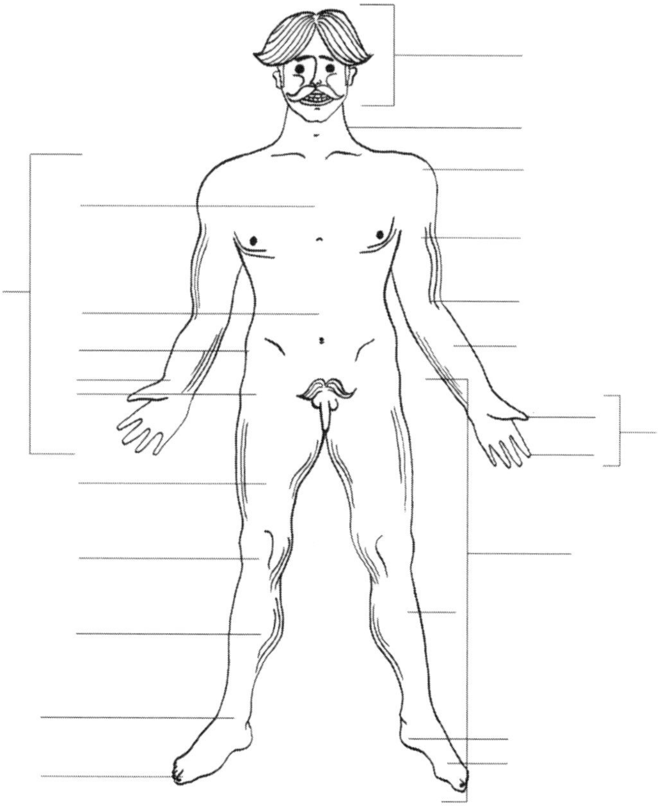

NURSING IN ACTION

At the emergency room...
Doctor: Nurse Robbins could you come over here a moment? Could you look after this patient? He fell off his motorbike and has got cuts, abrasions and **bruises** pretty much everywhere. Luckily, nothing's broken; he was only wearing jeans and a tee-shirt. He's lucky to be alive!
Nurse Robbins: Right, let me have a look at you – well there are some pretty **nasty grazes** on your ankles, shoulders, knees and elbows, and there's a **deep** cut on your eyebrow that'll probably need a few **stitches**. The doctor'll do that when he comes back.
I'll just have to **clean** the **wound** and disinfect it – I'm afraid this is going to **sting** a little.
Later…
Nurse Robbins: Let me see those grazes. They're quite deep too; I'm just going to clean them, put on some antiseptic **ointment** to help them **heal** and **dress** them. Try to keep the **dressing** dry, and arrange for a community nurse to come to see you twice a week for the next two or three weeks to change the dressing and to make sure there's no infection.
Are you up to date with your anti-tetanus **jabs**?

Word list

bruise	ecchymose / contusion
nasty	méchant
graze	éraflure
deep	profond
stitch	point de suture
wound	plaie
(to) sting	piquer
ointment	pommade
(to) heal	cicatriser
(to) dress (a wound)	panser
dressing	pansement
jab	piqûre

VIDEO

Upper Limb Examinations

http://www.youtube.com/watch?v=BOK8TroYSU8

Script:
Begin the examination of the motor system by observing the patient's body position **at rest**, and during movement. Also watch for involuntary movements. Next, assess muscle characteristics, beginning with **muscle bulk**. To do this, carefully inspect the muscles of the shoulders, arms, hands, thighs and legs, noting any atrophy. Then evaluate the patient's

muscle tone or resistance to **passive stretch**. Encourage the patient to relax, then take one hand in yours, and while **supporting** the elbow, **flex** and extend the patient's fingers, wrist, elbow and shoulder in one coordinated movement. The patient's arms should move easily and **smoothly** with little resistance. Repeat on the other side. To assess muscle tone in the legs, extend the patient's leg at the knee and move the foot up and down at the ankle. Note the patient's resistance to your movements. Assess muscle strength; use force compatible with the patient's strength. Usually, the patient's dominant side is stronger than the non-dominant side. Begin by testing flexion and extension at the elbow by having the patient **pull** and **push** against your hand. Next, test extension of the wrist. Now, test the patient's **grip**. Cross your middle and index fingers to protect them. Then, ask the patient to **squeeze** as hard as possible while you try to **remove** your fingers. Normally, you should have trouble removing them. Continue testing muscle strength by asking the patient to turn his palm down and **spread** his fingers. Check abduction by trying to force them together. Then, test opposition of the thumb. To do this, ask the patient to try to touch the **tip** of his little finger with the thumb while you resist the movement.

Word list

at rest	au repos
muscle bulk	volume musculaire
muscle tone	tonus musculaire
passive stretch	étirement passif
(to) support	soutenir
(to) flex	fléchir
smoothly	sans à-coups / en douceur
(to) pull	tirer
(to) push	pousser
grip	force de préhension
(to) squeeze	serrer
(to) remove	retirer / dégager
(to) spread	écarter
tip	bout / extrémité

HOW TO... GIVE SIMPLE INSTRUCTIONS?

To give instructions, use **the infinitive without to (V)**.

In the negative, use the structure **don't + V**.

Sequencing words are used to link the various instructions: *first, first of all, now, then, after that, next, finally...*

Ex. In order to examine a patient's knee reflexes, you need to give the following instructions: **First, take off** your shoes and trousers. **Now**, **sit** on the examination table. **Let** your legs hang over the edge of the table. **Relax**. **Don't think** about your legs.

EXERCISES

1. Match the instructions with the reasons given on the right.

1. Open your mouth and say ah !	a. I'm going to check your balance.
2. Take off your clothes and lie down on the examination table.	b. I'm going to check your visual acuity.
3. Close your eyes and stand on one leg.	c. I'm going to check your back.
4. Bend over and touch your toes.	d. I'm going to check your abdomen.
5. Follow my finger with your eyes. Don't move your head.	e. I'm going to check your throat.
6. Put your hand over your left eye and read the letters on the screen.	f. I'm going to check your ocular motor function.
7. Give me your wrist.	g. I'm going to check your pulse.

2. Translate the following sentences.

1. Quand je l'ai examiné, il avait une énorme ecchymose sur l'épaule droite.
2. Aura-t-il besoin de points de suture au menton ?
3. Serrez mes deux doigts aussi fort que vous le pouvez.
4. Mettez de la pommade tous les jours sur votre plaie.
5. N'écartez pas les doigts. Je veux vous observer au repos.
6. Ne retirez pas votre main pendant que je vous pique.

DO IT YOURSELF

Pair work: **Student 1**: Look at the picture above and describe the position of a part of the body.
Student 2: Say what part of the body it is without looking at the picture.

Ex. **Student 1**: It is located between the arm and the forearm.
Student 2: The elbow is between the arm and the forearm.

Chapter 5

HISTORY TAKING / L'INTERROGATOIRE DU PATIENT

BUILD YOUR VOCABULARY

present(ing) complaint	What's brought you to our clinic? What seems to be the trouble? ...
history of present illness	What kind of pain is it? When did you first notice these symptoms? ...
past history	Have you ever been hospitalised? Are you taking any treatment at the moment? ...
family history	Are both your parents alive and well? Does anyone else in your family suffer from this problem? ...
social history	Do you drink / smoke / do any sport...? Have you travelled abroad recently? ...
occupational history	What is your job? Are you in contact with any toxic substances? ...

NURSING IN ACTION

A consultation at the outpatients' department...
Nurse: Good morning Mr. Johnston. My name is Nurse Simpson.
Mr. Johnston: Good morning, nurse.
Nurse: Could you tell me a little bit more about your **headache**?
Mr. Johnston: Yes, of course.
Nurse: When did it begin?
Mr. Johnston: About eight days ago, but it's been getting worse, and over the last couple of days, it's been **unbearable**.
Nurse: Does the headache keep you **awake** at night?
Mr. Johnston: It disturbs my sleep, but I do manage to sleep a little.
Nurse: Have you taken anything for it?
Mr. Johnston: Yes, I tried **OTC painkillers**, you know, aspirin and paracetamol, but they didn't do much, I'm afraid.
Nurse: I see, and can you describe the headache?
Mr. Johnston: Yes it's a **throbbing** headache all over the head.

Nurse: Is it worse at any particular time of day?
Mr. Johnston: Yes, it's generally worse at the end of the day.
Nurse: I'd like to ask you about your family history. Are your parents alive and well?
Mr. Johnston: My mother is **fine**, but my father died of a **stroke** some years ago.
Nurse: I see, and can you tell me what type of stroke it was?
Mr. Johnston: I'm not sure; it happened so suddenly. I'll have to check with the hospital.
Nurse: Tell me, Mr. Johnston, are you taking any medication at the moment for high blood pressure, for example?
Mr. Johnston: No, nothing – I've always been pretty healthy.
Nurse: And what about your job, Mr. Johnston, have you been under pressure recently?
Mr. Johnston: Well, we've all been under pressure over the last few weeks. They're talking about **relocation** and **redundancies**, so we're all a bit worried.
Nurse: Right, Mr Johnston. Would you take off your shirt? I'd like you to lie down on the couch. I'm going to check your vital signs.

Word list

headache	mal de tête / céphalée
unbearable	insupportable
awake	éveillé
OTC (over the counter)	en vente libre
painkiller	antidouleur / antalgique
throbbing	pulsatile
fine	bien / en bonne forme
stroke	attaque (cérébrale)
relocation	délocalisation
redundancies	licenciements

VIDEO

Taking a patient's history

http://www.youtube.com/watch?v=vALxC4Rqx3E

Script:
Nurse: Good morning!
Patient: Good morning!
Nurse: Could you please **state** your name and your birth date?
Patient: Why are you asking me this?
Nurse: Well, I just want to make sure you are who I think you are.
Patient: That's a good idea! Ron Jones, December 15th, 1955.
Nurse: OK, and this is really just a **safety check** just to make sure I've got the correct patient, and I do. My name's Sue and I'm one of the nurses here.
Patient: Pleased to meet you
Nurse: Thank you! Er… I'm gonna just be asking you a few questions, a bit of a history, and I may be taking notes, it's just about that. So what brings you to our clinic today?
Patient: I've got a **cough**, well I've had a cough for a while now, but this past week, it seems to be getting worse. And I'm coughing stuff up.
Nurse: Some stuff, can you tell me about **the stuff you're coughing up** or the **sputum** you're **bringing up**?
Patient: It seems yellowish, but maybe sometimes **greenish-looking**.

Nurse: And how are you feeling generally overall?
Patient: Well I feel a bit tired all the time.
Nurse: OK. Are you having any fever or **chills**?
Patient: No.
Nurse: No. Are you on any medications?
Patient: Yes, I had been taking some antibiotics. They didn't seem to do much so I stopped taking them.
Nurse: OK! Well I'm just gonna give you a little information: antibiotics work best when you take the whole **dosage**. If you start and stop them, the bacteria might not be killed and then it can come back and be a little bit stronger. It's one of the medications when you should take the whole dose. And it's usually only seven or ten days at a time but you should take all of it.
Patient: Oh I didn't know that. Thanks for the information.
Nurse: Oh no problem! Back to your cough, are you a smoker?
Patient: Yes I've smoked for a long time.
Nurse: Can you tell me how many years of smoking that is?
Patient: Er… two packs a day, just about.
Nurse: And for how long?
Patient: Thirty-five years now.
Nurse: Have you ever thought about quitting?
Patient: Yes but that's really hard now.
Nurse: Yes I've heard that it is! I haven't experienced that but… I have some information on a smokers' **helpline**, would you like to see that?
Patient: Sure! What have I got to lose?
Nurse: OK! Well I'll give that to you before you leave. I know you told me you don't have a fever, but I would like to take your blood pressure, **pulse**, your vital signs, just before the doctor comes to see you, so is that OK with you?
Patient: Sure!
Nurse: And I'd like to listen to your chest as well. Ok? Well, I'll get that ready.

Word list

(to) state	indiquer
safety check	précaution
cough	toux
the stuff you are coughing up	ce que vous crachez
sputum	expectoration
(to) bring up	cracher
greenish-looking	d'aspect verdâtre
chills	frissons
dosage	posologie
helpline	centre d'assistance téléphonique
pulse	pouls

HOW TO... GIVE COMPLEX INSTRUCTIONS?

To be less direct and more tactful, **modal verbs** are occasionally used:
Would you take off your shirt, please?

Could you lie down on the examination table?
Will you remove your glasses, please?
I'd like you to take a deep breath.
I want you to push as hard as you can.

EXERCISES

1. Transform the following simple instructions into more tactful ones, using a different expression each time.

Ex. Close your eyes.
Will you close your eyes, please?

1. Bend over.
2. Stand on one leg.
3. Open your mouth.
4. Lie on your stomach.
5. Take off your shoes and socks.

2. Put the following words in the right order to form correct sentences.

1. have / feeling / you / how / been / today?
2. to / to / your / I / would / listen / like / chest.
3. it / at / of / any / worse / time / is / particular / day?
4. the / are / medication / moment / you / at / taking / any?
5. you / your / keep / does / night / headache / at / awake?
6. few / been / pressure / we've / the / under / over / weeks / last.
7. trouble / seems / to / what / be / the?
8. did / the / when / come / pain / on / exactly?

DO IT YOURSELF

Pair work: Use the following cues to continue the following history taking by asking questions (**student 1**) and answering in full sentences (**student 2**).

Ex. nausea / 5 days
Student 1: What's brought you along today?
Student 2: I've been feeling nauseous.
Student 1: When did it start?
Student 2: It started 5 days ago...

weight loss (4 kg) / vomiting / fever / diarrhoea / six or seven times a day / blood on the toilet paper/ type of pain (colicky) / location of pain (low abdomen) / first time / Burkina Faso / local food / local water / vaccinations / past operations (appendectomy at age eleven) / alcohol.

Chapter 6

THE SKELETAL SYSTEM / LE SYSTEME SQUELETTIQUE

BUILD YOUR VOCABULARY

skeleton	**squelette**
bone	os
cranium / skull	crâne
maxilla / upper jaw	maxillaire / mâchoire supérieure
mandible / lower jaw	mandibule / mâchoire inférieure
zygomatic bone / cheek bone	os zygomatique / pommette
scapula / shoulder blade	omoplate
clavicle / collarbone	clavicule
humerus / funny bone	humérus
ulna	cubitus
radius	radius
spine / backbone / spinal column	colonne vertébrale
rib	côte
sternum / breast bone	sternum
(cervical, thoracic, lumbar) vertebra	vertèbre (cervicale, thoracique,
(vertebrae)	lombaire)
pelvis	(vertèbres)
sacrum	bassin
ilium	sacrum
ischium	ilion
femur / thigh bone	ischion
patella / kneecap	fémur
tibia / shin bone	rotule
fibula / calf bone	tibia
calcaneus / calcaneum / heel bone	péroné
	calcanéum

NURSING IN ACTION

At the outpatient department...
Nurse: What's brought you along ?
Young man: Well, I think I've broken my ankle.
Nurse: First of all, could you tell me your name and address please?
Young man: Yes, it's Daniel Carter, and I live at 36, Gladstone road here in Brighton.
Nurse: And how old are you, Daniel?
Daniel: 23.
Nurse: Right, what happened?

Daniel: Well I was playing football on Saturday afternoon and I fell in a tackle and **injured** my ankle. It didn't seem too bad at first; the coach put the magic **sponge** on it, and I carried on playing for a few minutes, but then I had to stop; it was **hurting** too much.
Nurse: Why didn't you come to the hospital **straight away**?
Daniel: Well, the coach **bandaged it up**, and after the game we had a couple of beers and it felt O.K, so I thought it was just **twisted** or **sprained**.
Nurse: So, why have you come now?
Daniel: When I took the bandage off this morning, it was black and blue, very **painful**, and my foot was **swollen**, so I thought I had better get it **checked out.**
Nurse: Have you got any insurance for accidents that happen when you play football?
Daniel: No, I haven't.
Nurse: Have you told your employer that you're here?
Daniel: I'm **between jobs** at the moment.
Nurse: Well we'll need to get that ankle **X-rayed**, and the doctor will see you afterwards. I'll get a wheelchair for you and I'll get a health assistant to take you to the X-ray unit.
Daniel: Thanks.

Word list

(to) injure	blesser / se faire mal à
sponge	éponge
(to) hurt	faire mal
straight away	immédiatement
(to) bandage up	bander / mettre un bandage
(to) twist	tordre
(to) sprain	faire une entorse
painful	douloureux
swollen	enflé
(to) check out	vérifier / examiner
between jobs	en recherche d'emploi
(to) X-ray	faire une radio

VIDEO

The Skeletal System

http://www.youtube.com/watch?v=hkwAR8yjWAQ

Script:
The skeletal system is a **framework of bones** within your body whose arrangement determines how your body moves. The **shape** of the individual bones and the ways that they **fit together** allow you to stand and walk, and determine how the different parts of your body move.
Your spine is the central column that supports your body's **weight**. It is a **stack** of small bones called vertebrae. These bones are connected by joints which allow them to move a little in relation to one another. At the top of the spine, the first two vertebrae support your skull. The upper bone is called the atlas, after the mythical Greek **god** who **holds up** the **earth**. The second vertebra is called the axis. It is the joint between the atlas and your skull that allows you to move your head up and down.
A different joint between the atlas and the axis allows you to rotate your head from side to side.

The next group of vertebrae supports the bones of your **shoulder girdle** and the bones of your ribs. Rib bones form a cage that protects the **soft tissues** of your **heart** and **lungs**. Your ribs are **loosely** joined to your breastbone in a way that allows the entire structure to move as you **breathe**. **Below** the ribs, your spinal vertebrae are larger and stronger. These bones carry all the weight of your upper body. All the vertebrae are connected by joints that allow them to work together.

Word list

framework of bones	structure osseuse
shape	forme
(to) fit together	s'articuler
weight	poids
stack	empilement
god	dieu
(to) hold up	soutenir
earth	la terre
shoulder girdle	ceinture scapulaire
soft tissues	tissus mous
heart	cœur
lung	poumon
loosely	assez librement
(to) breathe	respirer
below	en dessous de

HOW TO... REFER TO THE PAST AND / OR THE PRESENT?

When referring to an event that **took place or that started in the past**:

- if the focus is on the present, use the **present perfect**.

Ex. Well, I think **I've broken** my ankle. (I think is is broken now)

- if the focus is on a past context, use the **simple past**.

Ex. After the game **last Saturday**, we **had** a couple of beers.

EXERCISES

1. Put the verbs in brackets in the right tense (simple past or present perfect).

1. I (take) Mr Smith's blood pressure ten minutes ago, and it (be) a bit high.
2. The nurse already (show) the patient to his room.
3. At what time (arrive) the patient this morning?
4. He (break) his back when he (fall) down the stairs.
5. Last night, the elderly patient (have) a stroke.
6. Where's my stethoscope? You (see) it anywhere?

2. Write the names of the following bones.

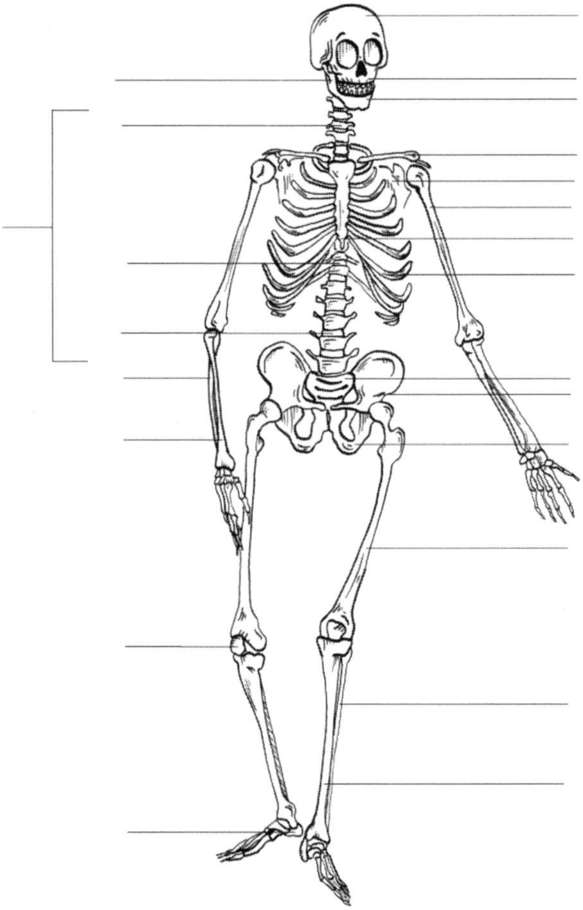

3. Here are the medical names of bones. Give the everyday English equivalent.

1. scapula
2. patella
3. tibia
4. maxilla
5. mandible
6. femur
7. clavicle
8. humerus
9. zygomatic bone
10. sternum
11. calcaneus

DO IT YOURSELF

Pair work: **Student 1** is looking for a paediatric nurse to hire; you ask questions to the nurse applying for the job. Use the table below to ask and answer questions. **Student 2** is a nurse applying for a job; use the table in **File 1** (p. 161) at the end of the book to ask and answer questions.

Ex. **Student 1:** Have you ever worked in a paediatric ward?
Student 2: Yes, I worked in a paediatric ward for seven months...

STUDENT 1
Experience in paediatric ward?
Reason for leaving previous position?
Reason for wanting the position?
Favourite part of the job?
Most hated part of job?
£22,000 / year
47 hours / week
6 am to 2pm
2 pm to 10 pm
10 pm to 6 am
...

Chapter 7

THE PATIENT'S ROOM / LA CHAMBRE DU PATIENT

BUILD YOUR VOCABULARY

Put the following words in the picture below:
armchair / bedside table / blanket / brush / comb / cup / cupboard / curtain / drawer / locker / napkin / pillow / sheet / towel / washbasin / washcloth

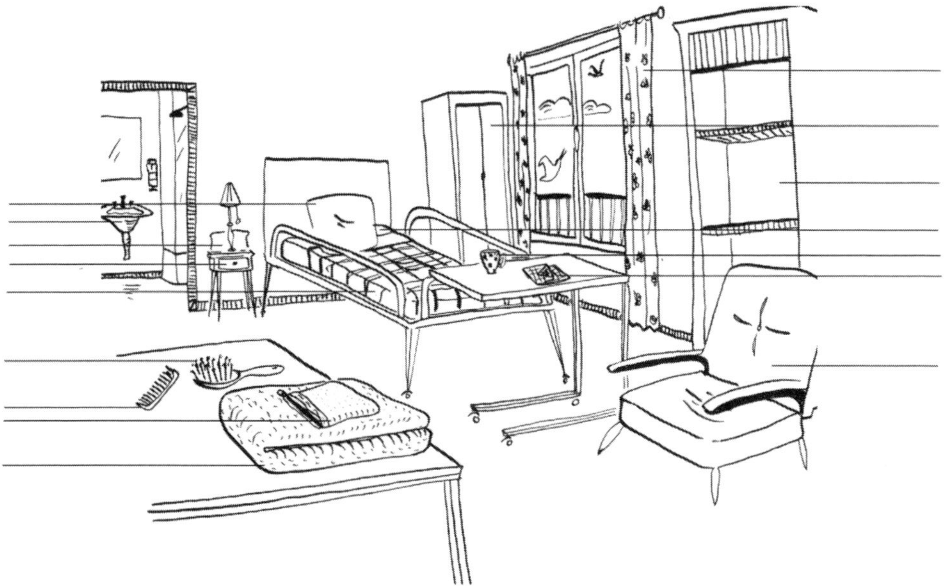

NURSING IN ACTION

In the patient's room...
Nurse: Here's your room; let me just explain one or two things.
As you can see, you have your own private bathroom and shower, and you can use these when you need to. Of course, after the operation, you won't be able to have a shower for **at least** four days, so a nurse will come to see you every day to take care of your personal

hygiene. And if you need to go to the toilet, just press the **call button** next to your bed, and someone will come very quickly.
After the operation, you may feel some **discomfort**, or even pain. Again, if you need a painkiller, press the call button.
You can put your clothes and **personal belongings** in the **wardrobe** and the bedside table. There's a drawer for your **bits and pieces**, hair brush, **make up and the like**. The hospital will provide towels and **soap**, but you will need to have your own **toothpaste**, shampoo and other **toiletries**. Have you brought your **dressing gown**?
Patient: Yes, I have; it's in my **suitcase**.
Nurse: Good.
Patient: What about visiting times? When can my children come to see me?
Nurse: Well, there are **no hard and fast rules**, but it's best if they come in the middle of the morning or the middle of the afternoon, because most of the treatments have been given and patient care has been **completed** then.
If these times don't **suit**, which is often the case for people who have to work, we do allow visits between 6.30 and 8 o'clock in the evening, but visitors mustn't make too much noise so as not to disturb other patients.
Coming back to your room, there's a television, but we only have the main **channels**, I'm afraid: BBC 1 and 2, and ITV.
Patient: That doesn't matter; I don't watch TV very often, and when I do, I only watch BBC1.
Nurse: Well, if you like to read in bed, there's a bedside lamp. The **switch** is just here.
Patient: Thank you very much; I'm sure I'll be very comfortable.
Nurse: Well, I'll let you **settle in**. And don't forget, if you need anything, just press the call button. The doctor will come to see you tomorrow morning. Oh yes, I forgot to mention, meal times are 7 in the morning, 12 noon and 6 in the evening.

Word list

at least	au moins
call button	sonnette
discomfort	(sensation de) gêne
personal belongings	effets personnels
wardrobe	armoire
bits and pieces	affaires personnelles
make up	maquillage
and the like	et autres
soap	savon
toothpaste	dentifrice
toiletries	articles de toilette
dressing gown	robe de chambre
suitcase	valise
no hard and fast rules	pas de règles absolues
(to) complete	terminer
(to) suit	convenir
channel	chaîne (de télévision)
switch	interrupteur
(to) settle in	s'installer

VIDEO

The Patient's Room

http://www.youtube.com/watch?v=EaU2CMucFPI

Script:

Journalist: Spacious, private patient rooms are the **cornerstones** of patient center design at Sacred Heart at Riverbend. The rooms include a **twin-size day bed** for a **loved one** to stay **overnight**.

Lola Fritz: Friends and family are really important to the patient's **healing process**. And we want to make sure that we **provide** a very comfortable, welcoming place for them in the patient's room.

Journalist: Research indicates that patients not only prefer private rooms, but also that patients are more likely to **share** sensitive health information with their **caregiver** in a private room. In addition, these quieter rooms **cut down on** the number of distractions caregivers face at the bedside. We've even moved the patient medication inside the private room, allowing caregivers to have the patient medication and a computer with the patient's electronic **medical record** together in a **non-disruptive** environment.

Lola Fritz: We want the nurses to be **focused on** giving the medication, the right medication to their patients, so we're gonna move the medications inside the room where they really can focus on that and avoid the distractions.

Journalist: To **prevent injuries** from **falls**, many of the private rooms also feature **ceiling lifts** to assist our patients as they get out of bed.

Lola Fritz: Ceiling lifts allow the caregivers to move the patients without pulling and **tugging** on them, so it's much more comfortable for the patient.

Journalist: Ensuring patients' safety, promoting family **involvement**, and creating a comfortable and private environment for the patients to **heal**, just a few of the reasons why the best care comes from the heart. Sacred Heart Medical Center at Riverbend.

Word list

cornerstone	pierre angulaire
twin-size day bed	canapé d'appoint deux places
a loved one	un être cher
overnight	pour la nuit
healing process	guérison
(to) provide	fournir
(to) share	partager
caregiver (US)	accompagnant / aidant
(to) cut down on	réduire
medical record	dossier médical
non-disruptive	calme / non perturbant
(to) focus on	se concentrer sur
(to) prevent	prévenir / empêcher
injury	blessure
fall	chute
ceiling lift	lève-malade
(to) tug	tirer (fort)
involvement	implication
(to) heal	guérir

HOW TO... TELL THE TIME?

It is important to distinguish between two systems:

1. The 12-hour system

The expression **o'clock** may be used to refer to a complete hour.

Ex. My appointment is at 10 (**o'clock**) in the morning.

For the first 30 minutes, the preposition **past** is used between the minutes and the hour.

Ex. 10.20 = twenty **past** ten
6.15 = **a quarter past** six
2.30 = **half past** two

From the half hour onwards, the preposition **to** is used between the minutes that remain and the next hour.

Ex. 8.40 = twenty **to** nine
9.45 = **a quarter to** ten

In this system, if the number of minutes is not a multiple of five, the word **minutes** must be used.

Ex. 7.22 = twenty-two **minutes** past seven

Unless the context is clear, it is necessary to mention whether it is the morning (am = ante meridiem) or the afternoon (pm = post meridiem).

Ex. The flight leaves London at **11 am** and arrives in Los Angeles at **3 pm** local time.

When it is 12 o'clock, you can specify **12 noon, noon, midday** (= midi), or **midnight** (= minuit).

2. The 24-hour system

It is based on the digital clock. The time is read from left to right.

Ex. 10.20 = **ten twenty**
6.15 = **six fifteen**
2.30 = **two thirty**
7.22 = **seven twenty-two**
13.04 = **thirteen O four**

EXERCISES

1.Translate the following sentences.

1. Vous pouvez mettre vos effets personnels dans l'armoire située à gauche de la porte.
2. Le lève-malade permet à l'infirmier de lever le malade plus facilement.
3. Vous aurez besoin des articles de toilette suivants : du shampoing, du dentifrice et du savon.
4. Pour appeler l'infirmière, il suffit d'appuyer sur la sonnette.
5. D'après son dossier médical, cette patiente s'est blessée en faisant une chute dans sa salle de bain.

2. Unscramble the words and match them with the definitions.

1. atrucins	You use it to clean your teeth.
2. htosubrhot	You sleep with your head on it.
3. rewdra	You use it to keep warm in bed.
4. ctubonaltl	You close them for privacy.
5. lketbna	You keep your bits and pieces in it.
6. willop	You use it to call a nurse.
7. usacites	From one day to the next.
8. gothenriv	You put your clothes in it when you go to hospital.

DO IT YOURSELF

Pair work:
Student 1 is a nurse.
Student 2 is a patient just admitted to the hospital who wants to know when...

- medication is given
- the doctor comes to visit
- visiting times are
- breakfast is
- lunch is
- dinner is
- vital signs are checked
- the bed bath is given
- ...

Chapter 8

ASSESSING PAIN / L'EVALUATION DE LA DOULEUR

BUILD YOUR VOCABULARY

Put the following words in the picture below:
cheeks / chin / ears / eyebrows / eyelashes / eyelids / eyes / forehead / hair / lips / moustache / mouth / nose / nostrils / teeth (one tooth) / tongue / wrinkles

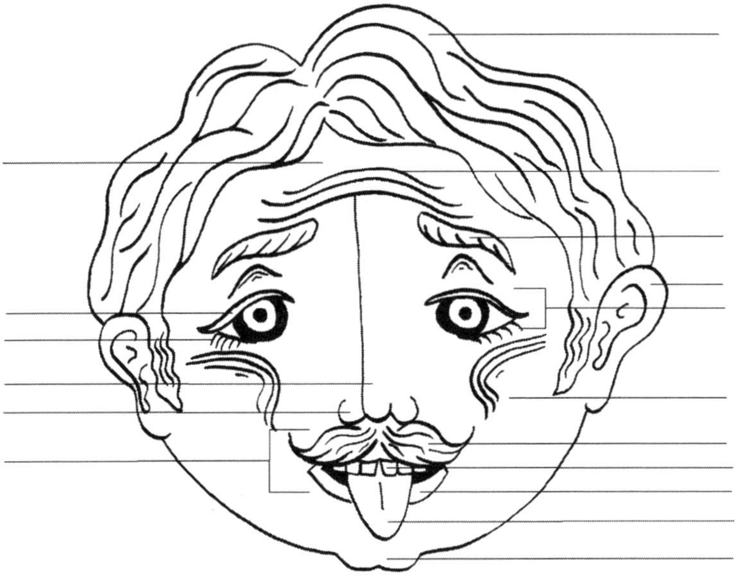

NURSING IN ACTION

At the nurses' station…
Senior nurse: One of the most difficult things to **deal with** in nursing is pain **management**. There are various reasons. **First of all**, not all patients can **bear** the same degree of pain. So, even though the level of pain might be the same - for example, the pain caused by a broken collarbone - some patients will **hardly** complain at all, while others will be **writhing in agony**.

Student nurse: What do we have to do then, give the same treatment to all of the patients with a broken collarbone, or **tailor** the treatment to the individual?
Senior nurse: This is the reason we have the VAS for pain assessment. That is the Visual Analogue **Scale**. Patients can use it to express the **amount** of pain they are experiencing, and treatment must be given in accordance with the scale. As you can see, scores range from 0 to 10, and with treatment, we **aim to** reach a score of three.
Student nurse: I remember reading about the placebo effect in the management of pain; is it true that sugar pills can help patients feel better?
Senior nurse: As I said, pain is very subjective; people react differently, so you have to **play it by ear** a little bit. Give the patient an analgesic and see how he reacts. If necessary, increase the dose or change to a **stronger** drug. You'll **eventually** develop a sort of feeling for the amount of pain **relief** you need to give.
Anyway, to come back to the problems of pain management, you may find yourself with very young **infants**, or mentally-handicapped patients, who can't understand the pain scale, and you have to judge the degree of pain by **carefully** observing them. A patient in extreme pain will be **moaning** or **crying**, hardly moving at all. In cases like, this you need to give a **powerful** analgesic. Then **keep an eye on** them to see if they become more relaxed; they may not **smile**, but they look calm when the pain **subsides**.
Student nurse: Are there any other ways of knowing if the pain relief has been effective?
Senior nurse: Well, you may see the blood pressure or the pulse fall. Usually, breathing will **slow down**: people in pain tend to breathe in fast, **shallow breaths**, but you can usually tell just by looking at the patient's facial expression.

Pain scale

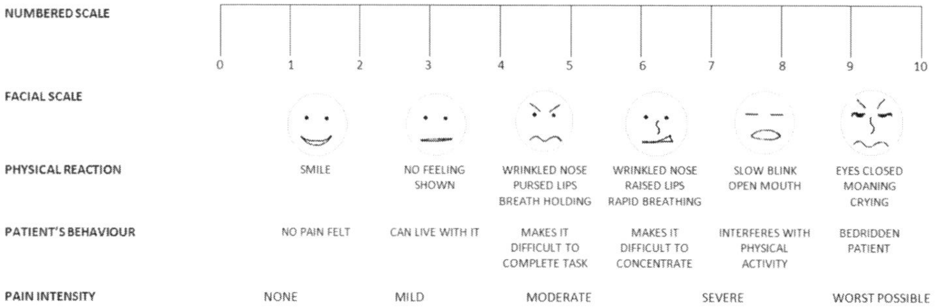

Word list

pain	douleur
(to) deal with	gérer / maîtriser
management	prise en charge
first of all	tout d'abord
(to) bear	supporter / tolérer
hardly	à peine / guère
(to) writhe in agony	se tordre de douleur
(to) tailor	adapter
scale	échelle
amount	quantité
(to) aim to	viser à / avoir pour objectif
(to) play it by ear	se fier à son instinct
strong	fort
eventually	finalement

relief	soulagement
anyway	quoi qu'il en soit
infant	nourrisson / bébé
carefully	attentivement / soigneusement
(to) moan	gémir / geindre
(to) cry	pleurer
powerful	puissant
(to) keep an eye on	surveiller
(to) smile	sourire
(to) subside	s'atténuer
(to) slow down	ralentir
shallow	peu profond
breath	respiration

VIDEO

Spain performs full face transplant

http://www.youtube.com/watch?v=elDDC9cpW-8

Script:
Journalist: This is a computer-generated image of how the patient's face looked before **surgery**. The unnamed young man lost his face in an accident. He could only breathe and be **fed** through tubes. Now he has a new nose, skin, jaws, cheekbone, teeth and other **features**. The remarkable operation to attach the new face took a thirty-member Spanish medical team twenty-four hours to **perform**.
Dr Joan Pere Barret: The patient asked to see himself one week after the surgery, and he reacted very calmly and with satisfaction. And when we asked him, in writing, because we communicate with writing and gestures, he said he was very **grateful** and satisfied.
Journalist: The hospital says the surgery was **carried out** in **late March**.
Dr Joan Pere Barret: He absolutely does not look like the donor patient, and I think that's important for society to know in terms of future donations of faces that there's no such danger of this.
Journalist: The world's first partial face transplant was carried out on Isabelle Dinoire in France in 2005. After the surgery, Dinoire **struggled** with the psychological challenges of **getting used to** her new different face. This Spanish operation is the first known full face transplant. The patient **is expected** to **remain** in hospital for two months.

Word list

surgery	opération chirurgicale
(to) feed (fed, fed)	alimenter
features	traits / caractéristiques
(to) perform	pratiquer / réaliser
grateful	reconnaissant
(to) carry out	pratiquer / réaliser
in late March	fin mars
(to) struggle	lutter / se débattre avec
(to) get used to	s'habituer à
(to) be expected to	être censé
(to) remain	rester

HOW TO... EXPRESS INTENSITY?

To express intensity or degree, you can use the following **adverbs**.
They are usually placed **before the adjective, the verb, or the past participle** they modify.
almost, nearly, barely, hardly, slightly, a little, a bit, mildly, quite, rather, enough, increasingly, far, highly, too, very....

Ex. This rate is **highly** (= fortement) variable.
I **barely** (= à peine) know this new patient.

Pay attention to the adverb **enough**; it always comes **after the adjective**.
Ex. The patient isn't **strong enough** (= pas assez fort / trop faible) to be transferred.

EXERCISES

1. Translate the following sentences.
1. Ouvrez la bouche et tirez la langue.
2. Les rides sur son front montrent qu'il a passé la soixantaine.
3. L'opération chirurgicale a été pratiquée fin juillet.
4. Le patient est censé rester au lit car la douleur est extrêmement sévère.
5. La douleur est légère. Elle n'entrave pas mon activité physique.
6. Sa respiration est de plus en plus rapide.

2. Fill in the blanks with one of the intensifiers above.
1. Could you speak _______ louder, please? I can _______ hear you.
2. Mr Smith is _____ weak to walk on his own.
3. The patient isn't warm _______. He needs another blanket.
4. Mrs James is _______ cured. She will soon be able to leave the hospital.
5. The disabled child is becoming _______ dependent on his parents.
6. She is _______ _______ old to live on her own.
7. I'm getting bored. The programme is only _______ interesting.

DO IT YOURSELF

Pair work: **Student 1** prepares four comprehension questions on the first half of the Nursing in Action text.
Student 2 answers them.
And vice-versa for the second half.

Ex. Student 1: What is one of the most difficult things to deal with in nursing?
Student 2: It is pain management.

Chapter 9

THE CARDIOVASCULAR SYSTEM / LE SYSTEME CARDIOVASCULAIRE

BUILD YOUR VOCABULARY

Put the following words in the picture below:

arch of aorta / ascending aorta / descending aorta / atrium (pl. atria) / coronary artery / inferior vena cava / myocardium / pulmonary artery / pulmonary trunk / pulmonary vein / superior vena cava / ventricle

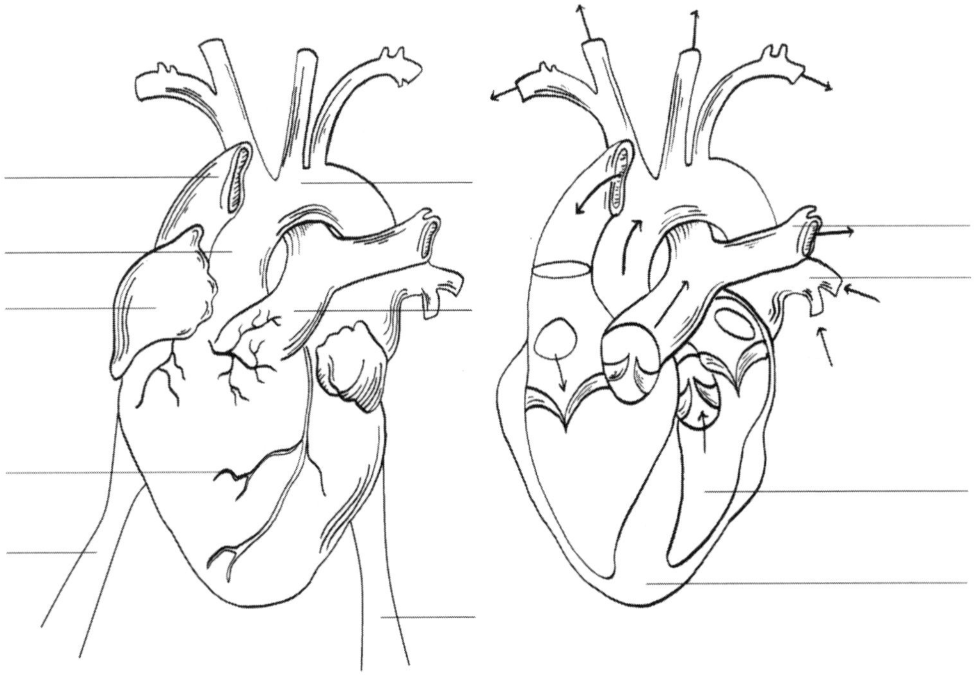

NURSING IN ACTION

At the cardiology consulting room.
The nurse has already noted down the patient's name, age and date of birth, and now focuses on the specific reasons for the consultation...
Nurse: Mrs Houghton. I'd like to get some details before you see Professor Cotton for the examination. First of all, you said you came because you have a pain in your chest.
Mrs Houghton: Yes, that's right.
Nurse: Could you describe the pain for me?
Mrs Houghton: Yes, it's a very severe pain and it **comes on** all of a sudden without **warning**, and I can't breathe – it's very **frightening**. It **feels like** my chest is all **constricted**.
Nurse: I see. And can you tell me exactly where it is?
Mrs Houghton: It's **right in the middle** here, under my breastbone, but sometimes it **spreads** to my left shoulder.
Nurse: How often do you have these pains?
Mrs Houghton: Well, it used to be very rare, but they're becoming more and more frequent, about **once** or **twice** a month, and more painful. That's why I thought I'**d better** have it checked, and my doctor said I should come and see you.
Nurse: Yes, **by the sounds of things**, I think that was the **right** thing to do. Professor Cotton is going to examine your heart. First of all, he'll do an **ECG** to see where the problem is, and then you'll be taken along to the cath lab for **a procedure** called a coronary angiography – he has to check your coronary arteries to make sure they're not **clogged up**. And if they are, he may insert a stent; it's a sort of metallic **device** that expands to open up your arteries to make the blood **flow** more easily.
Mrs Houghton: **Oh dear**, it sounds serious.
Nurse: Don't **worry**, Mrs Houghton, it's a **fairly** routine procedure and Professor Cotton is one of the best cardiologists in the country.
Mrs Houghton: I suppose you'll have to **put me to sleep**?
Nurse: No, not at all – we have to put a catheter, a sort of **thin** tube, into an artery in your thigh and then push it along up to your heart. It only needs a **local anaesthetic** where we insert the catheter. If everything goes well, it will take less than an hour, and as I told you on the phone, we have to keep you in overnight to make sure there's no **bleeding**.
Mrs Houghton: Oh dear, I'm not sure I like the idea of being awake.
Nurse: Don't worry, Mrs Houghton, I'll be there to talk to you and make sure you're comfortable.

Word list

(to) come on	survenir
warning	avertissement
frightening	effrayant
(to) feel like	avoir l'impression que
constricted	comprimé
right in the middle	en plein milieu
(to) spread	se propager
once	une fois

twice	deux fois
(you) had better	(vous) feriez mieux
by the sounds of things	d'après ce que vous en dîtes
right	bon, juste
ECG (GB)	ECG
procedure	intervention
clogged up	obstrué, bouché
device	dispositif / appareil
(to) flow	circuler, couler
Oh dear	Mon dieu
(to) worry	s'inquiéter
fairly	assez, plutôt
(to) put to sleep	endormir
thin	fin / mince
local anaesthetic	anesthésiant local
bleeding	hémorragie / saignement

VIDEO

Pacemaker for the heart

http://www.youtube.com/watch?v=B0UhT66qojM

Script:
Harry Smith: In this morning's HealthWatch, we look at a new device designed to warn us of **heart attacks sooner** rather than later. Our doctor Jennifer Ashton has details. Good morning!
Dr. Jennifer Ashton: Good morning to you, Harry. Each year, more than a million Americans have had a heart attack and a third of them will **die** even before getting to the hospital. Now the chances of **survival** increase every second **saved** in getting treatment. And now, a first alert system, something like **'OnStar'** for the heart, could mean the difference between **life** and **death**.
In the middle of the night, without warning, forty-two-year-old Lisa Hulce had a massive heart attack.
Lisa Hulce: I had extreme nausea, and then my arms and legs got **numb** and **tingly**.
A cardiac nurse educator, Lisa didn't recognize her own symptoms.
Lisa Hulce: I was **gasping for air**. I couldn't even explain what was going on.
Her husband ran next door for help and an ambulance **rushed** her **to** the hospital.
Husband: I believe I hold the park record for running in, **barefoot**, in **underwear**.
Lisa is lucky to be **alive**. But with a family history of heart disease, she knew it could happen again.
Lisa Hulce: It was really kind of a **scary** experience.
A year ago, she became one of the first patients to be implanted with a pacemaker-like device that constantly **monitors** her heart's **EKG** or electrical activity, looking for changes that can **occur** even before a heart attack's first symptoms. Any problems, a **hand-held** unit sounds an alarm.

Word list

heart attack	crise cardiaque
sooner	plus tôt
(to) die	mourir
survival	survie
(to) save	gagner
Onstar	système de sécurité 'Onstar'
life	la vie
death	la mort
numb	engourdi
tingly	qui picote / qui donne des fourmillements
(to) gasp for air	suffoquer / haleter
(to) rush	se précipiter
barefoot	nu-pieds
underwear	sous-vêtements
alive	en vie
scary	effrayant / terrifiant
(to) monitor	surveiller
EKG (US)	ECG
(to) occur	survenir
hand-held	portatif

HOW TO... QUALIFY PAIN?

To express types and degrees of pain, you can use the following adjectives:

acute (aiguë)
burning (sensation de brûlure)
chronic (chronique)
constrictive (constrictive)
crushing (sensation d'écrasement)
dull (sourde)
excruciating (atroce)
localised (locale)
mild (discrète)
moderate (moyenne / modérée)
radiating (qui irradie)
sharp (vive / intense)
shooting (lancinante)
stabbing (en coup de poignard)
stinging (sensation de décharge électrique)
throbbing (pulsatile)
unbearable (intolérable)

EXERCISES

1. Translate the following sentences.

1. L'artère est bouchée ; nous ferions mieux de poser un stent.
2. Le patient s'est plaint de douleurs de poitrine atroces qui sont apparues tout d'un coup sans avertissement.
3. Le vieil homme, qui a été transporté en urgence à l'hôpital, est toujours en vie grâce aux soins prodigués par les urgentistes.
4. Lorsque le médecin est arrivé, elle était allongée par terre, en train de suffoquer.
5. Ne vous inquiétez pas. La douleur est bien trop discrète. Vous n'allez pas avoir une crise cardiaque.
6. D'après ce que j'ai compris, c'est une question de vie ou de mort. Il faut envoyer le patient au bloc immédiatement.

2. Look at the pictures below and choose the adjective that best describes the type or degree of pain that is represented.

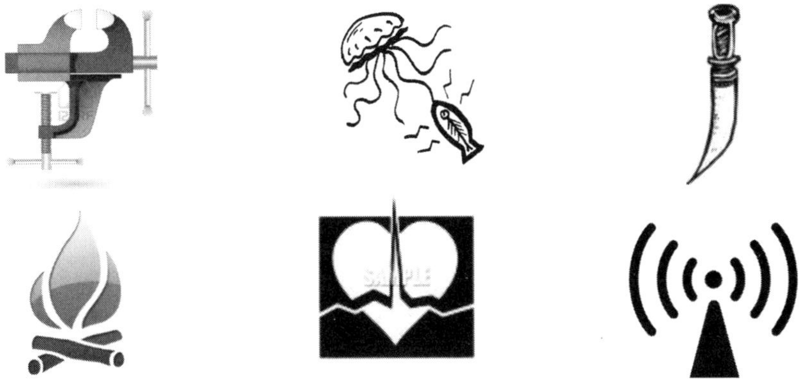

DO IT YOURSELF

Pair work: Split crossword puzzle

Student 1 looks at the crossword below, and **student 2** looks at the crossword in **File 2** (p.161).

Student 1 asks **Student 2** for definitions or explanations of missing words.

Student 2 gives the definitions or the explanations without using the missing word.

Student 1 tries to find the word.

And vice versa, one word at a time.

This activity will give you the opportunity to practice the alphabet.

	a	b	c	d	e	f	g	h	i	j	k	l	m	n	o	p	q	r
1			H			E	C	G									F	
2	F	-	E	-	-		-						-				L	
3	O		A		M	Y	O	C	A	R	D	I	U	M			O	
4	A	-	R	-	-		-		T		-		-		V		W	
5	M		T		-		-		R		-		-	-	E	-	S	-
6				B	L	E	E	D	I	N	G		-		N			
7				-			-		U		S	T	E	N	T			
8		T		-		-			M	I			-		R		-	
9	C	H	R	O	N	I	C			-			-	-	I	-	-	
10		I		-		-		N	O	S	E				C		-	
11		G				-				-			V	A	L	V	E	
12		H	E	A	L	E	D		-	-	-	-			E		-	
13						-				-								

Ex.

Student 1: What is a-2 across?
Student 2: It means "to have a sensation".
Student 1: Is it "to feel"?
Student 2: That's right, but in the third person.
Student 1: "feels"
Student 2: That's right! What is c-1 down?
...

Chapter 10

PAIN MANAGEMENT / LA PRISE EN CHARGE DE LA DOULEUR

BUILD YOUR VOCABULARY

pain	douleur
suffering	souffrance
suffer from	souffrir de
pain clinic	centre anti-douleur
pain assessment	évaluation de la douleur
pain relief	soulagement de la douleur
(to) dull	atténuer
(to) relieve	soulager
(to) alleviate	soulager
(to) soothe	calmer
(to) ease	calmer
treatment	traitement
painkiller / analgesic	antidouleur / analgésique
physiotherapy (GB) / physical therapy (US)	kinésithérapie

NURSING IN ACTION

Two nurses are having a discussion during the coffee break (Yes, they do have coffee breaks!)...

Nurse Johnson: What a job – it's incredible how much **lifting** and **carrying** we have to do in a day!

Nurse Greenwood: I know, last year I had terrible **trouble** with my back. Every time I tried to lift anything I had a terrible shooting pain right down to my ankle.

Nurse Johnson: That sounds terrible; I know **low-back pain** is a very **common** problem for nurses. We hear about **slipped discs**, lumbago, sciatica and even vertebral fractures in some of the older staff. Who did you go to see?

Nurse Greenwood: I **put up with** it for a couple of months, and then it was so bad, I went to see Doctor Constantine in Rheumatology. He found out what the problem was **right away** – sciatica. Apparently it was the sciatic nerve **root** that was **pinched** in the lumbar vertebrae. The disc was **slightly** herniated, and sometimes the nerve got **trapped**. It was horrible.

Nurse Johnson: So, what did he give you for it?

Nurse Greenwood: Well he gave me some anti-inflammatory drugs, and he prescribed a few **sessions** of physiotherapy. He also told me to try swimming or cycling to **balance** the muscles in my back and strengthen them a bit. Oh yes, and he gave me something to relax

my muscles as well. I had to take it at night, just before I went to bed. I must say, it **worked wonders**. If I'd known it would have worked so quickly, I would have gone to see him earlier.
Nurse Johnson: What about the physiotherapy?
Nurse Greenwood: The physiotherapist was great; she gave me some exercises to do, and she massaged my spine. It really alleviated the pain. She said that I was right to act quickly before the **damage** was too serious.
Nurse Johnson: And did you **take up** a sport?
Nurse Greenwood: Yes, I took out my old bicycle and cleaned it up, and now I come to work on it. It's great; I **save** money on **petrol**, my back is better and I feel much healthier. I can recommend it.
Nurse Johnson: The health and safety people at the hospital have organized a few training sessions on how to lift **properly** without injuring your back; perhaps I'd better go to one.

Word list

(to) lift	soulever
(to) carry	porter
trouble	ennuis / problèmes
low-back pain	douleur lombaire
common	fréquent
slipped disc	hernie discale
(to) put up with	supporter / faire avec
right away	immédiatement
root	racine
pinched	pincé / coincé
slightly	légèrement
trapped	coincé / comprimé
session	séance
(to) balance	équilibrer
(to) work wonders	faire des miracles
damage	dégâts
(to) take up	commencer / se mettre à
(to) save	économiser
petrol	essence
properly	correctement

VIDEO

Chronic pain

http://www.youtube.com/watch?v=4Be9gRv75hU&feature=related

Script:
Journalist: **According to** the Centers for Disease Control, one in ten Americans have had pain for one year or more, and many people can't work, they lose their jobs, they become depressed. CBS 4 **health** specialist Dr Sean Kenniff says there are plenty of options out there. But the key is for patients to **commit** to finding a treatment that works for them.
Dr. Sean Kenniff: Thirty-nine-year old Tom Carlin has tried several treatment options for pain that began more than 10 years ago.

Tom Carlin: They did physical therapy, you know, ultrasound, massage therapy, and all sorts of **stuff**.
Dr. Sean Kenniff: After years of **searching for** relief, he found a doctor who specializes in pain management and a treatment that works.
Tom Carlin: I found that the nerve blocks work very well for me.
Dr. Sean Kenniff: Dr Bruce Mann says the **goal** is to give patients like Carlin some relief so they can rebuild **weakened** muscles.
Dr Bruce Mann: **Significantly** reduce the pain so that the patient can tolerate, maybe, physical therapy and **therefore** maintain and restore function, strength, and mobility.
Mary Ballantine: I had six major back surgeries, five in the last three years.
Dr. Sean Kenniff: Several back surgeries **failed** to alleviate Mary Ballantine's pain. The forty-year old has been suffering for nearly three decades. When conventional treatments failed, Dr Edward Fankowski who specializes in interventional pain management recommended she try a pain stimulator.
Dr Edward Fankowski: It works almost like a pacemaker in a sense that it stimulates the spine, using electricity the same way a pacemaker stimulates the heart.
Dr. Sean Kenniff: Once inserted into the lower back, **leads** are connected to the area causing pain. Patients can control the amount of electrical stimulation through a **remote device**. These stimulators have been around for years but recent **improvements** make the battery last much longer, **up to** 10 years.
Dr Edward Fankowski: The goal of that is to try and block the electrical impulses that go along the **spinal cord** and block them before they get to the **brain**.
Dr. Sean Kenniff: She can now work regularly and enjoy life a whole lot more.
Mary Ballantine: Yeah, I can play with my granddaughter. Yeah, it helps.
Dr. Sean Kenniff: Now, it's not unusual for pain specialists to try several different modalities on a patient before finally finding something that works. And **by the way**, **even** when patients do find something that works, it doesn't always take away their pain one hundred percent, but it usually does **allow** them to **improve** their quality of life.

Word list

according to	selon
health	santé
(to) commit to	s'engager à
stuff	trucs / choses
(to) search for	chercher
goal	but
(to) weaken	affaiblir
significantly	de façon significative
therefore	donc / par conséquent
(to) fail	échouer / ne pas réussir à
leads	dérivations
remote device	télécommande
improvement	amélioration
up to	jusqu'à
spinal cord	moelle épinière
brain	cerveau
by the way	d'ailleurs / à ce sujet
even	même
(to) allow	permettre
(to) improve	améliorer

HOW TO... EXPRESS DURATION?

Questions that begin with **how long** and the preposition **for** are used to express length of time.

Ex. **How long** have you been ill?
I've been feeling sick **for** a week or so.

The expression **since when?** and the preposition **since** refer to a starting point (a date, a day, a year, a period in the past...)

Ex. I haven't been feeling well.
Since when?
Since last weekend

For answers the question **(for) how long?**
During answers the question **when?**

Ex. The operation went on **for** three hours.
During the operation, they decided to remove his appendix.

EXERCISES

1. Fill in these sentences with FOR, SINCE or DURING.

1. He hasn't been to the doctor ________ 1999.
2. I have quit smoking ________ four weeks now.
3. How long is your treatment? I have to take it ________ five days.
4. She has been suffering from her shoulder ________ her car accident.
5. She's been having insulin injections ________ she was 17.
6. The vaccine will be efficient ________ eight months.
7. You can't take analgesics ________ more than seven days.
8. She contracted a nosocomial infection _______ her hospital stay.

2. Translate these sentences into English.

1. Je ne supporte plus ces douleurs lombaires.
2. Le but de cette séance est de renforcer les muscles affaiblis.
3. Cela fait des années que ce kinésithérapeute fait des miracles !
4. Tu portes trop de trucs, tu vas finir par avoir une hernie discale!
5. Ma santé s'est améliorée de façon significative depuis que je me suis engagé à suivre ce traitement.

DO IT YOURSELF

Pair work: **Student 1** is a patient suffering from ... and answers questions to the nurse.
Student 2 is a nurse trying to help a patient find a proper treatment by asking questions to the patient.

Ex.
Student 1: low-back pain / 4 months / lorry driver / analgesics
Student 2: What is your problem? / Since when? / How did it happen? / What is your job? / What treatment...?

- knee / one year / knee surgery / car accident / pain relief / ...
- headaches / sneezing / coughing / last spring / ...
- left shoulder / two weeks / factory worker / anti-inflammatory drugs / ...
- ankle / yesterday / dancing / ice / ...
- back / six months / secretary / physiotherapy / ...

Chapter 11

THE MAIN INTERNAL ORGANS / LES PRINCIPAUX ORGANES INTERNES

BUILD YOUR VOCABULARY

Put the following words in the picture below:

brain / bronchi / heart / large intestine / liver / lung / small intestine / spleen / stomach / trachea

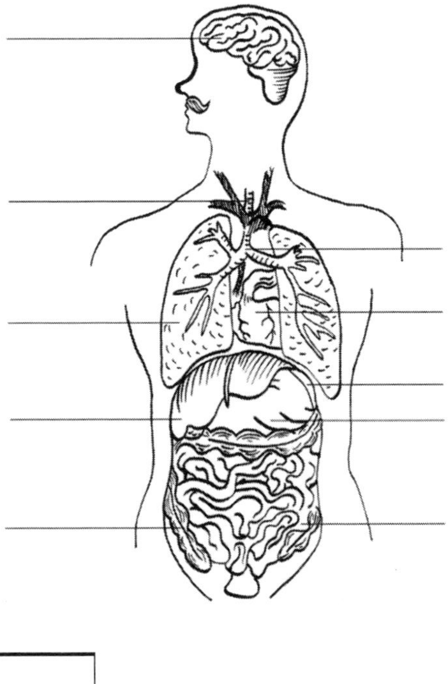

NURSING IN ACTION

*During the **induction course**, an instructor gives a talk about **organ donation**...*
Nurse instructor: During your years as nurses you'll be confronted with patients in very serious **predicaments**: accident victims, patients who have to have **kidney** dialysis 3 times a week, patients with **failure**, who can't even walk from one room in their house to

another, or patients with blood or lung diseases whose life is **hanging by a thread**. These are patients of all ages, from young children to **old-age pensioners**, but who all want to live as healthy a life as possible for as long as possible. Many of these patients could be **treated** or in some cases even **cured**, if they could receive a **donated** liver or kidney, or a bone **marrow** transplant.

And this is why I've come to talk to you today. It's all about carrying a **donor** card. I've carried one since I was a student like you, and over the years, my experience has convinced me that I made the right choice. On countless times, I've seen people in great physical and mental pain, people who had been in and out of hospital for years, with virtually no hope of a normal life, walk out of the hospital with a smile on their faces knowing that all of the suffering was over and knowing that they'd been given a second chance to enjoy life.

It's the greatest **gift** that you can give, and I **urge** you all to think about it, to talk to you loved ones and make the decision to help those in need.

And remember, one day you might need a blood transfusion or a transplant, and you will be very grateful for the **thoughtfulness** of others. It's true, we hear about cultivating organs and tissues from **stem cells**, and scientists are really making incredible progress, but it will be many years before organ donation is no longer necessary.

Well, I've said what I wanted to say, so do any of you have any questions?

Student nurse: If someone carries a donor card, can anyone in the family, for example, stop doctors from taking organs for transplantation?

Nurse Instructor: It's better to talk to your family and explain your decision and get their **agreement**. You have to put yourself in their shoes. They've just been told that a **daughter** or **brother** or **son** has died, and someone comes along to ask about taking their organs; it's not an easy situation, so it's best if they are prepared.

Student nurse: Does the **recipient** ever get to know who the donor was?

Nurse instructor: Generally speaking, donations are anonymous to **avoid** ethical **issues**.

Word list

induction course	stage d'accueil
organ donation	don d'organe
predicament	situation difficile
kidney	rein
failure	insuffisance / défaillance
(to) hang by a tread	tenir à un fil
old-age pensioner	retraité
(to) treat	traiter / soigner
(to) cure	guérir
(to) donate	donner
marrow	moelle
donor	donneur
gift	don / cadeau
(to) urge	exhorter / conseiller vivement
thoughtfulness	prévenance / bienveillance
stem cell	cellule souche
agreement	accord
daughter	fille
brother	frère
son	fils
recipient (US)	receveur
(to) avoid	éviter
issue	question

VIDEO

The importance of your vital organs

http://www.youtube.com/watch?v=-4OQ7FUczfA

Script:

Doctor 1: So let's **go through** these organs. You've got three really important organs. I'm gonna be the champion for the heart. This little **fist**-sized muscle mass is **truly** an **amazing** organ, **beats** a hundred thousand times a day. Two thousand **gallons** of **blood** a day. Without this, you don't have life.

Doctor 2: Yeah, but you also gotta have your lungs too, and that's what this is. This little **slice** of a lung and it's kind of a big **spongy** organ. You have two of them: one on the right, one on the left, and it's responsible for taking in oxygen and **getting rid of** carbon dioxide and other gases and exchanging them into your blood, and you know, when you **breathe in** and **out**, that happens about 12 to 20 times a minute. But what's really amazing about the lungs is all these **tiny** microscopic sacs in there, little air sacs called alveoli, and the total surface **area** of the lung is about the **size** of a tennis court, so pretty amazing.

Doctor 3: Of course, they got machines for both those things, right? Heart-and-lung machines. They don't have a machine for the brain at all. I love the brain. Not yet. Yeah, right, maybe one day.

Doctor 4: Isn't that kind of **biased** since you're a neurosurgeon?

Doctor 2: Yeah, you're a little biased.

Doctor 1: You said you didn't like the brain and you went into neurosurgery.

Doctor 3: I love the brain. This is the brain, and it's **actually** one of the most amazing organs, I think, and Fred has mentioned that, most of the blood from the heart goes to the brain, about twenty percent of all of the blood in the body goes here and over here the frontal lobe which is responsible for your **ability** to judge things, all your judgements. People who have damaged frontal lobes simply lose their judgement on the left side of the brain - this is the temporal lobe - this is the right side. On the left side, that's responsible for all of your language. Not only your ability to speak and write, but your ability to understand everything. Over here's your vision, back here, back here's your **cerebellum**, that's your **balance**; and on the **bottom** of your brain, you have the beginning of the **brain stem**. Without that, you can't coordinate your breathing, your **heart rate**. What are you without a brain? It's really nothing, it's amazing! This is the **outer layer**, called the dura, which we have to remove or cut through every time we perform an operation.

It's really an amazing thing.

Doctor 1: And the important thing is they are all **interlinked**. You can't live without any of these.

Word list

(to) go through	passer en revue
fist	poing
truly	véritablement
amazing	stupéfiant
(to) beat	battre

gallon	4,51 (GB) / 3,81 (US)
blood	sang
slice	tranche
spongy	spongieux
(to) get rid of	éliminer / se débarrasser de
(to) breathe in	inspirer
(to) breathe out	expirer
tiny	minuscule
area	aire / surface
size	taille
(to be) biased	manquer d'objectivité
actually	effectivement / en fait
ability	capacité
cerebellum	cervelet
balance	équilibre
bottom	partie inférieure / bas
brain stem	tronc cérébral
heart rate	fréquence cardiaque
outer	externe
layer	membrane / couche
(to be) interlinked	(être) lié

HOW TO ... REFER TO THE FUTURE?

To refer to the future, various verb forms are used:

Modal verbs	During your years as nurses you'**ll** be confronted with patients in very serious predicaments. That information **may** come in the next decade.
Modal phrases	I am afraid we **are going to** have to remove your left kidney. **I'm gonna** be the champion for the heart. It is difficult to know which cells **are likely to** turn deadly. I **have to** change this I.V. line this afternoon.
Reference to the present	She **is seeing** her doctor on Friday. The conference **starts** at 6 pm.

EXERCISES

1. Find the organs which correspond to the following definitions.

1. The large dark red organ in the upper part of the abdomen on the right side just beneath the diaphragm.
2. The large gland-like organ situated in the upper left part of the abdominal cavity.

3. The long tube-like structure where food is digested.
4. The two organs in the lumbar region that remove waste from the blood and secrete urine.
5. The organs of respiration lying on either side of the heart within the chest cavity.
6. The hollow muscular organ which receives the blood from the veins and propels it into the arteries.
7. The part of the central nervous system contained within the cranium.

2. Translate the following sentences.

1. Je vois l'infirmière en chef demain à 14h.
2. Le stage d'accueil commence à 10h.
3. Croyez-moi, il va guérir rapidement.
4. Les enfants, il faudra éviter de courir dans les couloirs de l'hôpital !
5. Votre don d'organe va certainement sauver la vie d'un enfant.
6. Il se peut que votre fille et votre fils aient la même maladie que vous.

DO IT YOURSELF

Pair work: Here is your programme for the week. **Student 1** explains to **student 2**, who missed the presentation, what he or she will be doing (**use various expressions from the grammar notes above**).

Programme for the coming week.

Monday: Talk and practical work: how to set up an I.V. line. (practical work on **dummies**).
Tuesday: Dressing burn wounds – lesson and visit to the burns unit of the hospital (groups of four – visit: 1 hour approx.).
Wednesday: 2 groups alternate morning and afternoon: either - moving patients to avoid bedsores, techniques to minimize discomfort to the patient and avoid excessive effort for nurses – Or – bed-bathing techniques – the dos and don'ts – talk and practice with patients at the old people's home.
Thursday: Either: visit to the regional trauma unit (optional) – this will take the whole day so bring a picnic lunch. - bus leaves at 08:00 and returns at 17:30. Register with administrative assistant for 1st year students,
Or: additional practice on I.V. lines.
Friday: Managing pain – Morning: lesson on pain mechanisms, different types of pain and pain assessment. Afternoon: introduction to pain relief medication, uses, doses, effects and side effects.

Chapter 12

MEDICAL INSTRUMENTS AND HOSPITAL HYGIENE / INSTRUMENTS MEDICAUX ET HYGIENE HOSPITALIERE

BUILD YOUR VOCABULARY

Put the following words in the picture below:

autoclave / blood pressure gauge / clamp / forceps / gloves / sticking tape / leads / sticking plaster / scalpel / scissors / staples / stethoscope / nail trimmer / compress / syringe / tray / tympanic thermometer / wipe

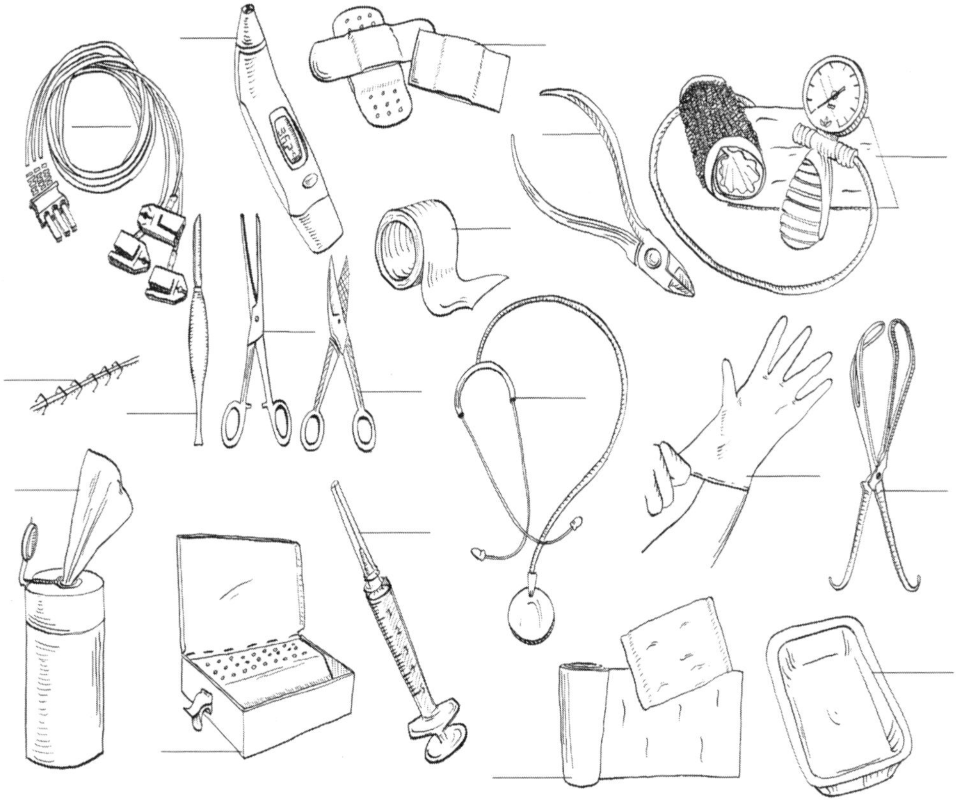

NURSING IN ACTION

An instructor is giving a talk to a group of student nurses at the outpatients' department...
Every day you have to make sure that the examination **cubicles** for outpatients are well stocked with the instruments and **supplies** that you or the doctors will need during a typical day. There's nothing worse than having a patient with a deep cut, for example, **lying** on the examination table, and then having to **hunt around** to get the things you need to treat him. It **wastes** precious time and gives a poor impression of the hospital and its staff.
This will be part of your job, so make sure you do it properly. In every cubicle, there is a checklist of the instruments such as **tweezers**, **stitch-cutters**, scissors, syringes, blood pressure cuffs, **probes** and thermometers that are used all the time, and **consumables** like disinfectant, sticking tape, gloves, **suture sets**, **gauze**, **cotton wool, swabs** etc.
So, wherever you're working, **find out** where the main store is and get to know the procedures for restocking the cubicles.
Most instruments are **packed** in sterile envelopes and these can only be used once. This means that after every patient, the instruments that have been used have to be **disposed of.** Syringes, for example, should be placed in a special container in the cubicle – you must never try to put the **cap** back on a syringe because you risk **pricking** yourself and infecting yourself with any disease that a patient may have. These are incinerated. Other instruments like scissors or forceps must be sent to the central sterilization unit so that they can be sterilized and used again. So, again, find out about the procedures to follow for the **disposal** of used instruments and hospital **waste**.

Word list

cubicle	box
supplies	fournitures
(to) lie	être allongé
(to) hunt around	chercher (partout)
(to) waste	gaspiller
tweezers	pince à épiler
stitch cutter	coupe-fil
probe	sonde
consumables	produits (de consommation)
suture set	boîte à suture
gauze	gaze
cotton wool	coton hydrophile
swab	compresse / écouvillon
(to) find out	chercher à savoir
(to) pack	emballer
(to) dispose (of)	jeter
cap	capuchon
(to) prick	piquer
disposal	élimination
waste	déchets

VIDEO

The decontamination process

http://www.youtube.com/watch?v=pZSX_xOllio&feature=related

Script:
In a **health care facility**, both you and your patient are at risk of coming into contact with disease causing microorganisms. This video presentation is **designed** to help you reduce the risks of disease within your workplace. While direct contact is generally **unavoidable**, we will focus on surface and instrument decontamination in medical office and ambulatory care **settings**. Disease can be transmitted from patient to patient, from patient to healthcare worker or from healthcare worker to healthcare worker. It can easily spread when given the right **set of** circumstances. Disease is reduced by decontaminating patient care equipment, instruments and work surfaces, as well as cleaning, **sanitizing** and disinfecting and sterilizing wherever pathogens may reside. The infection risk is reduced if the number of organisms is reduced. **Proper** cleaning, disinfection and sterilization procedures - **along with** practicing good hand hygiene - will reduce the risk of disease transmission to patients, visitors and employees. Decontamination is the general term used to describe the cleaning activities in the healthcare facility. Decontamination includes cleaning, disinfection and sterilization. Cleaning is the physical **removal** of **foreign** materials such as **soil** and blood from surfaces. Instrument cleaning removes microorganisms from surfaces and reduces the **soiled** layers that might interfere with the disinfection process later on. Disinfection is the decontamination process where most of the microbial population with the exception of spores is destroyed. A test accompanying this video will help your staff assess what they know about surface decontamination, how to prevent transmission of infection and provide a safe environment for patients and co-workers. Hand-washing, cleaning and disinfection are only one part of the control and elimination of disease. But they're probably the most **effective** and **inexpensive** processes.

Word list

health care facility	établissement de soins de santé
(to) design	concevoir
unavoidable	inévitable
settings	cadre / contexte / environnement
(a) set of	un ensemble de
(to) sanitize	aseptiser
proper	adéquat / correct
along with	ainsi que / accompagné de
removal	élimination
foreign	étranger
soil	terre / souillures
(to) soil	souiller
soiled	souillé
effective	efficace
inexpensive	peu coûteux / bon marché

HOW TO... EXPRESS METHOD AND GOAL?

By V-ing can be used to express manner, means and methods.

Ex. Disease is reduced **by decontaminating** patient care equipment.
Needlestick injuries can be avoided **by disposing** of used needles properly.

For V-ing can be used to express function.

Ex. A pair of forceps is a medical instrument **for compressing or grasping** tissue in surgical operations and **for handling** sterile dressing.

To + V can be used to express goal.

Ex. This video presentation is designed **to help** you reduce the risks of disease within your workplace.

EXERCISES

1. Translate the following sentences.

1. Vous pourrez améliorer votre anglais en apprenant le vocabulaire régulièrement.
2. Pour devenir infirmier diplômé d'état, vous devez faire trois années d'études.
3. Un scalpel est un petit couteau tranchant pour faire une incision.
4. Pour prendre la tension, vous avez besoin d'un tensiomètre.
5. Le stéthoscope est un appareil médical pour ausculter les poumons.
6. Vous éviterez le risque de contamination en vous lavant les mains régulièrement.

1. Find the instruments or consumables which correspond to the following definitions.

1. A medical instrument for compressing or grasping tissue in surgical operations and for handling sterile dressing.
2. A tool for picking up or handling small objects.
3. A device used to inject drugs into a vein or muscle, for example.
4. A piece of soft material used for cleaning wounds.
5. A dressing that can be stuck to the skin to protect a small wound or cut.
6. An instrument for measuring blood pressure in an artery.

DO IT YOURSELF

Pair work: Student 1 needs certain equipment or consumables to care for a patient and **student 2** says what is required. Use the vocabulary above.

Ex. **Student 1**: I want to take his temperature.
Student 2: Here's the thermometer.

Chapter 13

THE RESPIRATORY SYSTEM / LE SYSTEME RESPIRATOIRE

BUILD YOUR VOCABULARY

Put the following words in the picture below:

alveolus (pl alveoli) / bronchiole / bronchus (pl. bronchi) / diaphragm / larynx / lobes / lower airways / lungs / mouth / nasal cavity / nose / pleura / pleural cavity / throat / upper airways / trachea (windpipe)

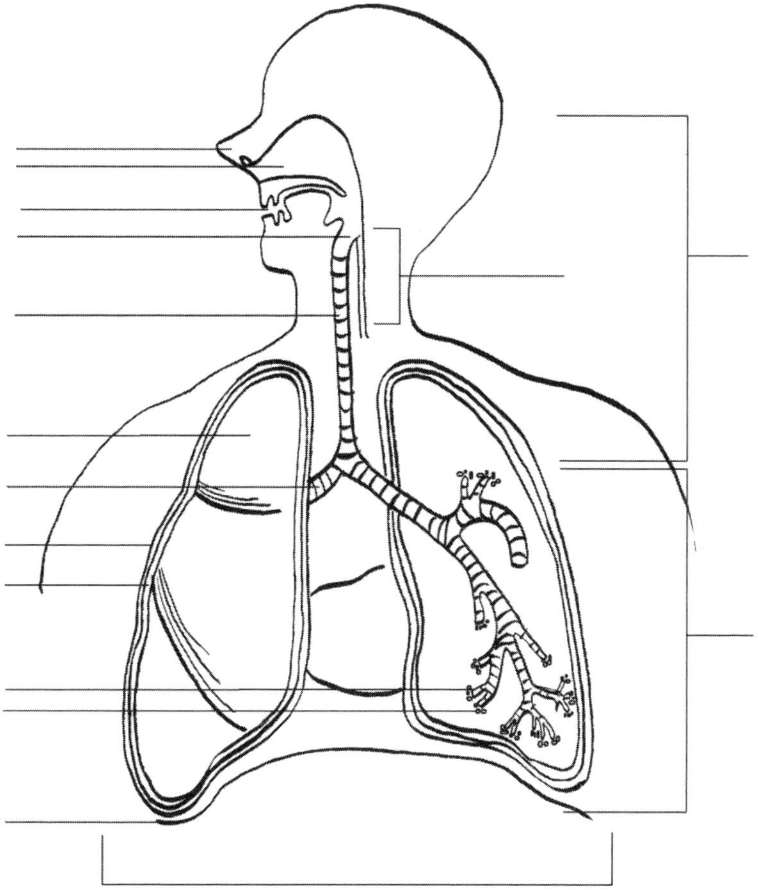

NURSING IN ACTION

At the pneumology department...
Senior nurse: Here in the pneumology department, we meet patients with all sorts of respiratory diseases, patients with asthma, pneumonia, lung cancer, pulmonary embolism or pneumothorax.
Student nurse: Excuse me, what's pneumothorax?
Senior nurse: This is when air gets into the **pleural space** and causes the lung to **collapse**.
Student nurse: Thank you.
Senior nurse: That's alright – don't hesitate to ask questions if there's anything you don't understand. Where was I? Oh yes, the most frequent examinations that we have to perform are pulmonary or **lung function tests**. In these tests we can measure various features of lung function, such as **peak airflow** and lung volume.
I'll show you how to use a **peak flow meter**, and then you can practice on each other.
Angela, could you come over here, please?
Before you start, you have to move the red indicator to its start position, here at the bottom of the scale.
Now, Angela, I'd like you to **take a deep breath**. Try to **fill** your lungs as much as possible, **hold your breath** for a moment while you close your lips as **tightly** as you can around the **mouthpiece**, and **blow** as hard and as fast as you can. Write down the position of the indicator – this is the peak flow.
You have to do the examination three times and **record** the highest of the three **readings** on the **daily record chart**.
Student nurse: What do we do if we have a patient who can't blow very hard?
Senior nurse: This happens all the time. Remember, these patients sometimes have very severe **respiratory distress** and they find it difficult just to breathe, so they just have to do what they can.
Student nurse: Do we have to change the mouthpiece after every examination?
Senior nurse: Yes, of course, these patients may have severe infectious diseases.
Student nurse: What do we do if there are very big differences between the readings?
Senior nurse: This doesn't happen very often; if you explain very carefully what the patient has to do, there are generally at least two that are fairly close together.

Word list

pleural space	cavité pleurale
(to) collapse	s'affaisser
lung function test	explorations fonctionnelles respiratoires
peak airflow	débit expiratoire de pointe
peak flow meter	débitmètre de pointe
(to) take a deep breath	inspirer profondément
(to) fill	remplir
(to) hold one's breath	retenir sa respiration
tightly	fermement
mouthpiece	embout
(to) blow	souffler
(to) record	relever / enregistrer

reading	relevé / mesure
daily record chart	feuille de suivi
respiratory distress	détresse respiratoire

VIDEO

Breathing

http://www.youtube.com/watch?v=sU_8juD3YzQ

Script:
During normal **breathing**, the air you inhale passes unobstructed down your trachea. This **sturdy** tube is **held** open by **rows** of C-shaped **bands** of cartilage. The open **end** of each C faces the esophagus, allowing the esophagus to open during **swallowing**. Air flowing down the trachea passes over **cilia**, epithelial cells with tiny hairs that **wave about** twenty times per second. These **sweep** more particles **out of** the air and trap them in a layer of **sticky** mucus that **coats** the trachea's **walls**. Cigarette smoke can paralyze these cilia, allowing these damaging particles to enter the lungs. Particles are **propelled** back upward by the cilia until they reach the esophagus. Then they are **swallowed** and disposed of by the digestive system. **Meanwhile**, air that has been cleaned, warmed and **moistened** continues down the trachea. Soon, the trachea divides into two smaller tubes: the bronchi. These tubes enter the lungs, then divide again and again until they are microscopic in size. Some of these are called bronchioles. Air travels along the bronchioles until they end in **grape-like clusters** of **air sacs**: the alveoli. These clusters **make up** the **inner** surface of your lungs. You have about 300 million alveoli in your lungs. Their combined **surface area** is about 70 **square meters**, some 600 square feet. Why such a large surface area? To **gather** enough oxygen from the air you breathe to **supply the needs** of all the trillions of cells in your body.

Word list

breathing	respiration
sturdy	robuste
(to) hold	maintenir
row	rangée
band	anneau
end	extrémité
swallowing	déglutition
cilia	cils
(to) wave	osciller
about	environ
(to) sweep out of	extraire de
sticky	visqueux
(to) coat	tapisser
wall	paroi
(to) propel	propulser
(to) swallow	avaler
meanwhile	pendant ce temps
(to) moisten	humidifier

grape-like	en forme de grappe
cluster	amas
air sac	alvéole / sac aérien
(to) make up	former / constituer
inner	interne
surface area	surface / aire
square meter	mètre carré
(to) gather	récupérer
(to) supply the needs	répondre aux besoins

HOW TO... USE RELATIVE PRONOUNS?

The relative pronoun **that** is used when the relative clause defines the antecedent (the word placed before it).

Ex. The most frequent examinations **that** we have to perform are pulmonary or lung function tests.

The relative pronoun **who** is used to refer to a person.

Ex. What do we do if we have a **patient who** can't blow very hard?

The relative pronoun **which** is used to refer to a thing, an animal, or an idea.

Ex. The **mouthpiece, which** has to be changed after every patient, must be fixed tightly to the peak flow meter.

The relative pronoun **what** is used when there is no antecedent. The French equivalent is often *ce que, ce dont, de quoi...*

Ex. If you explain very carefully **what** the patient has to do, there are generally at least two that are fairly close together.

EXERCISES

1. Translate the following sentences.

1. Ce relevé que j'ai pris la semaine dernière est plus bas que celui d'aujourd'hui. Cela montre que sa fonction pulmonaire s'améliore.
2. Il souffre de détresse respiratoire depuis plusieurs mois.
3. Inspirez profondément par les narines, retenez votre respiration quelques instants, puis expirez par la bouche.
4. Ces cils qui oscillent protègent la paroi de la trachée.
5. Est-ce que ça vous fait mal à la gorge quand vous toussez ?
6. Ces mucosités visqueuses bouchent les alvéoles et tapissent les bronches.
7. Les mesures notées dans sa feuille de suivi sont fausses.

2. Fill in the blanks with the right relative pronoun.

1. Doctor Johnson, ________ is a pneumologist, has just joined the department.
2. This patient must be sent to the ICU immediately, that is ________ I think.
3. The peak flow meter, ________ is used to measure the lung capacity of a patient, is easy to use.
4. We have lost the blood sample ________ Doctor Cooper asked for.
5. The hospital has just hired Nurse Foreman, ________ will be the new head nurse.
6. ________ you need to learn is how to dress a wound properly.

DO IT YOURSELF

Pair work: **Student 1** describes a part of the respiratory system.
Student 2 has to find the answer.
Exchange roles after each definition.

Ex. **Student 1**: It's part of your face, you use it to eat, swallow and breathe.
Student 2: It's my mouth!

Chapter 14

THE GASTROINTESTINAL SYSTEM / LE SYSTEME DIGESTIF

BUILD YOUR VOCABULARY

Put the following words in the picture below:

anus / large intestine (colon) / bowel / epiglottis / gallbladder / liver / oesophagus (gullet) / oral cavity / pancreas / rectum / salivary glands / small intestine / stomach / teeth (sg. tooth) / tongue

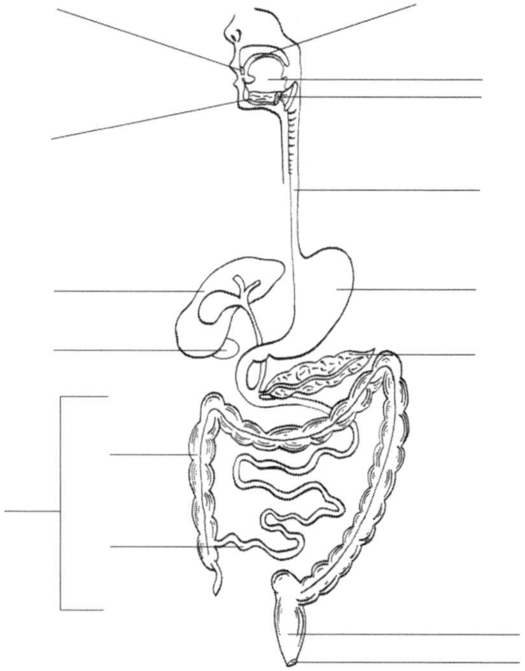

NURSING IN ACTION

During a ward visit...

Ward sister: One of the biggest problems in hospitals is feeding patients. Most patients can eat normal food, and so they are given the normal hospital meals made in the kitchens here.

This is one of the few hospitals where meals are prepared **on the premises**. Some patients, however, especially in intensive care, have to be fed through a nasogastric tube. The food arrives in **sealed** plastic **feeding bags**, and it's just a question of connecting the tube to the new bag.
Student nurse: How do we know when patients need feeding, when they are in a coma, for example?
Ward sister: Generally, we monitor **blood sugar,** blood **electrolytes,** and other parameters like **nitrogen** in the urine, and of course, a lot of research has been done about **nutrient** needs with regard to body weight and physical activity, so we know pretty well what a patient's needs are.
Student nurse: Do these patients need to go to the toilet like other patients?
Ward sister: Of course, the food in the bags is specially prepared so there is very little residue, but there is waste and this has to be dealt with. **Needless to say**, very sick patients can't go to the toilet and so they are **fitted with** collector bags.
To carry on, feeding is also very important in very **elderly** people because they **tend to** have lost their appetite, and very often they have difficulty **chewing** and swallowing. So, if you're not careful they'll hardly eat anything at all; that's why nurses have to **spend quite a lot of time** encouraging them to eat.
Student nurse: I suppose we have to spend quite a lot of time helping patients to go to the toilet or running around with **bedpans** and **bottles**.
Ward sister: You're right, it's a **time-consuming** part of the job, and as it's a very **sensitive issue**, you have to be very **understanding** and diplomatic, especially at first with new patients, but they get used to the routine very quickly.
What's more, in some diseases, or because of the treatments they're taking, patients may suffer from diarrhoea or constipation, so for patients who can go to the toilet, you may need to ask them about their **bowel movements**. "Were the **motions looser** than usual, or did you notice any blood or mucus on your **stools**, or did you have any bowel movements today, for example?" It's very important to be **aware** of these problems because patients may need treatment or a change of drugs.
Student nurse: Do we have to record all this information somewhere?
Ward sister: If the patient notices any changes in **bowel habits** or pain or blood, you must inform the ward sister, and she will take appropriate action.

Word list

on the premises	sur place / dans les locaux
sealed	scellé
feeding bag	poche d'alimentation
blood sugar	glycémie
electrolytes	ionogramme
nitrogen	azote
nutrient	nutriment
needless to say	cela va sans dire
fitted with	équipé de
elderly	âgé
(to) tend to	avoir tendance à
(to) chew	mâcher / mastiquer
(to) spend (time)	passer (du temps)
quite a lot of time	pas mal de temps
bedpan	bassin hygiénique
bottle	pistolet

time-consuming	chronophage
sensitive	sensible
understanding	compréhensif
bowel movement	mouvement intestinal / défécation
motions	selles
loose motions	selles diarrhéiques / peu consistantes
stools	selles
aware	conscient
bowel habits	habitude intestinale

VIDEO

Eating and digestion

http://www.youtube.com/watch?v=Z7xKYNz9AS0

Script:
In digestion, food is changed by the organs into a soluble form to be absorbed by the body. Food in the mouth is mixed with saliva. Saliva begins to dissolve the food as the teeth **grind** and cut it. Food is forced back into the throat (pharynx) by the tongue. Food in the pharynx stimulates the swallowing reflex. The larynx is pulled **upward** to meet the epiglottis and **seal off** the trachea. Food goes from the pharynx to the esophagus. Food moves down the esophagus by peristalsis. The peristaltic **wave** reaches the esophageal sphincter, and food enters the stomach. The unique muscular structure of the stomach **breaks up** the food into small pieces called chyme. Chyme exits through the pyloric sphincter into the duodenum of the small intestine. The major portion of absorption and digestion occurs in the small intestine. The **mucosa** secretes enzymes that supplement the digestive enzymes of the pancreas and liver. This completes the chemical process of digestion. The **walls** are covered with **villi** where nutrient absorption takes place. The structure of each **villus** contains a **capillary** and **lacteal** to **pick up** the digestive nutrients. The nutrients are now transported by the blood to all the **cells** of the body. The undigested food reaches the ileo-cecal valve and enters the large intestine or colon. The colon absorbs water, manufactures vitamins, produces mucus, and forms and expels **feces**. Mass peristalsis pushes the feces into the rectum, which stimulates the defecation reflex.

Word list

(to) grind	écraser / broyer
upward	vers le haut
(to) seal off	obstruer
wave	onde
(to) break up	décomposer
mucosa	muqueuse
villi (sg villus)	villosités
capillary	capillaire
lacteal	chylifère
(to) pick up	absorber
cell	cellule
feces	matières fécales / excréments

HOW TO... REFER TO ACTIVITIES?

The noun form of the verb (**V-ing**) is often used to refer to activities.

Ex. **Smoking** kills.
How do we know when patients need **feeding**?
Nurses have to spend quite a lot of time **encouraging** them to eat.
Always wash your hands before **examining** a patient.

EXERCISES

1. Find the parts of the body which correspond to the following definitions.

1. These are used to cut and crush the food before it is swallowed.
2. Large organ in the upper abdomen which secretes bile and cleans the blood.
3. The tube that connects the mouth to the stomach.
4. The large elongated gland lying behind the stomach between the spleen and duodenum.
5. A large sac between the oesophagus and the small intestine.
6. The pear-shaped pouch which serves as a storage reservoir for bile.

2. Translate the following sentences into English.

1. Passer du temps auprès des personnes âgées est une des activités des infirmiers.
2. Il est conseillé de bien mastiquer la nourriture avant de l'avaler
3. Les dents broient les aliments et l'estomac les décompose.
4. Il va sans dire que l'ionogramme est effectué dans les locaux de l'hôpital.
5. Les patients diabétiques doivent surveiller leur glycémie quotidiennement.
6. Après avoir mangé trop de fruits, il a eu des selles diarrhéiques.

DO IT YOURSELF

Pair work: Think of a few major activities a nurse has to do and describe them to your partner.

Ex. **Student 1**: First fill the syringe with the medical product, make sure there are no bubbles, then disinfect the skin with an antiseptic.
Student 2: Giving an injection / injecting a drug.

Chapter 15

THE GENITOURINARY SYSTEM / LE SYSTEME GENITO-URINAIRE

BUILD YOUR VOCABULARY

Put the following words in the pictures below (some words may be used twice):

bladder / cervix / kidney / ovary / penis / prostate / scrotum / spermatic cord / testicles = testes (sg. testis) / ureter / urethra / uterine tube = Fallopian tube / uterus = womb / vagina

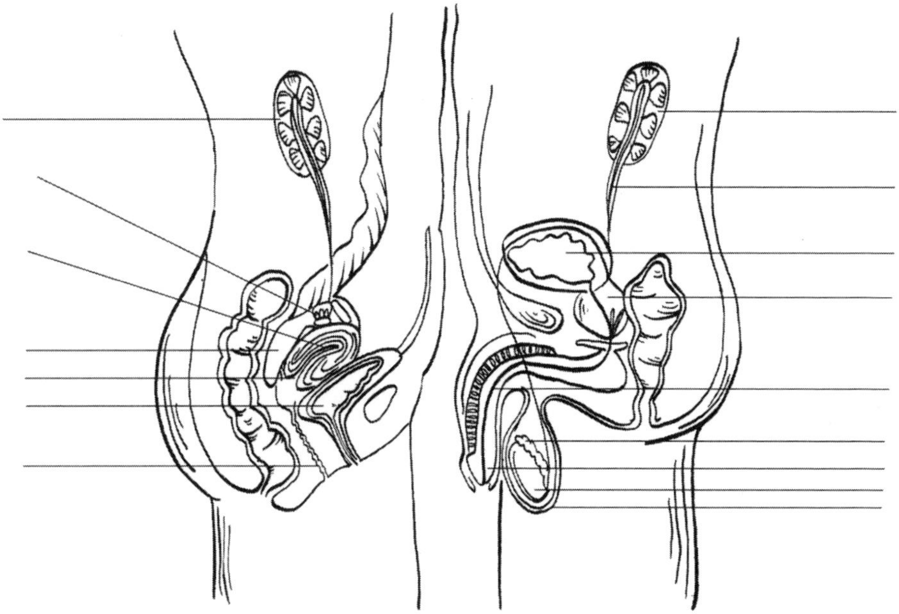

NURSING IN ACTION

Two student nurses at a patient's bedside...
Philip: It says on this **patient's chart** that the patient has **UTI**; what's that?
Sarah: Don't you remember we had a lesson on that a couple of days ago.
Philip: I must have missed it – I was **off sick** for three days last week. So, what is it?
Sarah: It **stands for** urinary tract infection. It's very common in **bedridden** patients, especially when they have a **urinary catheter**.

Philip: So what do we have to do when we have a patient with UTI?
Sarah: In fact, in most cases it's relatively easy to treat, a single dose of oral antibiotics generally **does the job**. But sometimes it can be quite difficult; it depends on where the infection is.
Philip: How do you mean?
Sarah: Well, if it's in the lower urinary tract, the urethra or the bladder, it's relatively benign, but if it's higher up and gets into the kidneys it can be quite dangerous. It can cause kidney failure and even sepsis if it's left untreated. It's the **leading cause** of death due to sepsis in hospitalized patients.
Philip: Wow, it's that serious!
Sarah: Yes it is, so you have to keep your eyes open for any signs of UTI.
Philip: What are the signs then?
Sarah: Well, first of all the patients may **complain about** needing to **pass water** more often and then pain or a burning sensation when they do. Then the urine may be particularly **smelly**, or may be **cloudy** or **bloody**.
Philip: Did they say anything about prevention?
Sarah: Patients with a risk of UTI should drink plenty of water to **flush out** the system, and cranberry juice is supposed to give pretty good protection because it makes the urine too acidic for **bacteria** to survive. Urine is supposed to be sterile, you know. Then we have to be scrupulously clean when we insert a urinary catheter, for example. Most of these infections are caused by bacteria that are found around the rectum. That's why women are advised to **wipe** from front to back and not vice-versa. Women, in fact, are far more likely to get a UTI.
Philip: I see. And how do we know if there is a serious infection?
Sarah: If it's bad, the patient may complain of nausea or vomiting or **dizziness**. There may be chills or fever or the patient may have pain in the back or the side or the abdomen.
Philip: Well, you've really learned your stuff. Could I make a photocopy of your notes for the lessons I missed?
Sarah: Sure, I'll bring them in tomorrow.
Philip: Thanks, you're a **pal**.

Word list

patient's chart	feuille de suivi
urinary tract infection (UTI)	infection urinaire
off sick	malade / arrêté
(to) stand for	signifier / vouloir dire
bedridden	alité / grabataire
urinary catheter	sonde urinaire
(to) do the job	faire l'affaire
leading cause	cause principale / première cause
(to) complain about / of	se plaindre de
(to) pass water	uriner
smelly	malodorant
cloudy	trouble
bloody (urine)	sang (dans les urines)
(to) flush out	nettoyer / rincer
bacteria (sg bacterium)	bactéries
(to) wipe	essuyer
dizziness	vertiges / étourdissements
pal	copain - copine / pote

VIDEO

Urassist

http://www.youtube.com/watch?v=bdaDLxhvKBA

Script:
The issues facing health care have become much more complex. The **shortage** of nursing personnel in America is creating challenges for **health care providers** concerned about patients' satisfaction. A significant amount of nursing time is devoted to **assisting** patients with the most common bodily function: the **means** to urinate. This is not only a time consuming nursing **task**, it can be an uncomfortable and sometimes difficult experience for patients. The use of bedpans and **urine bottles** often requires frequent attention from nursing personnel throughout the day. In a recent **survey**, one hospital indicated that nursing personnel can spend as much as 1.5 hours a day assisting patients with urination. **Reliance** on catheterization may put patients at risk for infection. Urinary tract infection or UTIs are the second most common hospital-induced infections occurring today. Additionally, **slip** and fall accidents affecting both patients and nurses frequently occur as a result of urine **spills** on the floor.
The **growing** need for health care to find more effective methods to control costs, save time and minimize health and **liability** risks, **sets the stage** for the **latest** technological advancement in urine collection and **storage**. Urassist is a unique **patented** urine collection and storage solution, providing an innovative alternative for health care facilities to improve nursing care and patient satisfaction. The automated system is easy for patients to use. First, instruct the patient to open the front door and Urassist automatically **turns on**.
Nurse: Open the door **gently**; you hear the pump come on…
Urassist fluid pump technology gently **draws** the urine **away** from the patients' body, minimizing odor, **leakage** and possible spills, as well as reducing unwanted **moisture**. Urassist includes collection cups for both male and female patients. Once finished, instruct the patient to simply replace the cup and close the door, which automatically shuts off the pump. Patients no longer need to call each time they have the **urge** to urinate.

Word list

shortage	pénurie
health care provider	personnel soignant
(to) assist	aider
a means	un moyen
task	tâche
urine bottle	pistolet
survey	enquête
reliance	dépendance
(to) slip	glisser
spill	flaque
growing	croissant
liability	responsabilité civile
(to) set the stage	planter le décor
latest	tout dernier
storage	stockage

patented	breveté
(to) turn on	se mettre en marche
gently	délicatement / doucement
(to) draw away	aspirer
leakage	fuite
moisture	humidité
urge	besoin pressant / impérieux

HOW TO... COMPARE?

Superiority is expressed as follows:
Ex. The pancreas is **smaller than** the kidney.
Patients feel **more comfortable** using Urassist.

Expressing degree:
Ex. The large intestine is **far shorter than** the small one.
Women, in fact, are **far more likely** to get a UTI.
The issues facing health care have become **much more complex**.

EXERCISES

1. Translate the following sentences into English.

1. Elle a glissé à cause d'une flaque d'urine et s'est cassé le poignet.
2. Les bassins hygiéniques brevetés utilisés dans les hôpitaux présentent rarement des problèmes de fuites et d'humidité.
3. Elle a du sang dans les urines depuis deux jours. Ce doit être une infection urinaire.
4. Le système est facile à utiliser pour les patients âgés.
5. Le patient se plaint de vertiges quand il se lève. Avez-vous vérifié sa feuille de suivi ?

2. Fill in the gaps with words taken from the lists above.

1. ICU _______ _______ Intensive Care Unit.
2. Hysterectomy is the removal of the _______.
3. This patient has been _______ _______ headache for several hours now.
4. After his accident he was _______ for a few months.
5. The _______ _______ of lung cancer is smoking.
6. A low level of blood sugar often causes _______.

DO IT YOURSELF

Pair work: **Student 1** gives three elements.
Student 2 makes a sentence using the comparative.

Ex. **Student 1:** burns / bruises (painful)
Student 2: Burns are far more painful than bruises.

1. liver / prostate (big)
2. X-ray / ECG (dangerous)
3. beta-blockers / aspirin (expensive)
4. teeth / tongue (hard)
5. ear infection / HIV (frequent)
6. UTI / men-women (often)

Deuxième année

S3-S4

Chapter 16

THE BLOOD: SETTING UP AN I.V. / LE SANG : MISE EN PLACE D'UNE PERFUSION

NURSING SKILLS: SETTING UP AN I.V.

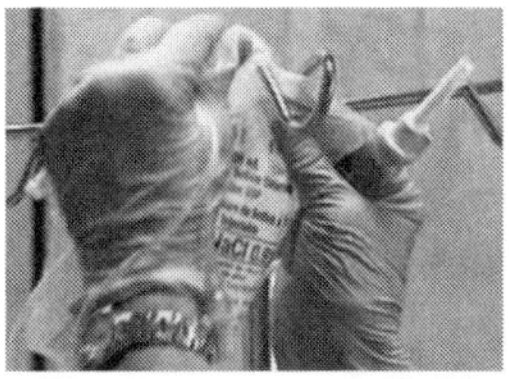

The intravenous fluid bag **hangs** at the bedside.

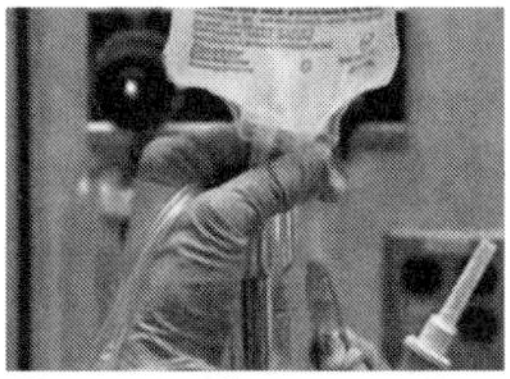

Remove the protective cap over the **tubing** insertion **spike**.

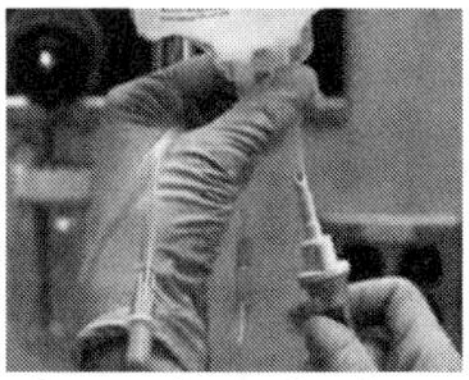

Insert the spike into the opening.

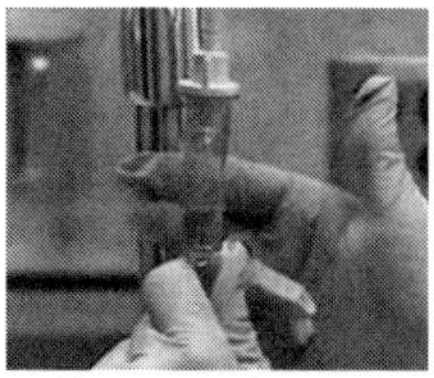

Squeeze the **drip chamber** until it is half **full**.

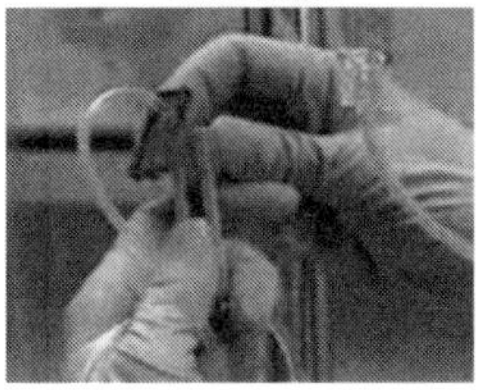

Unroll the **roller clamp** and keep it lower than the chamber.

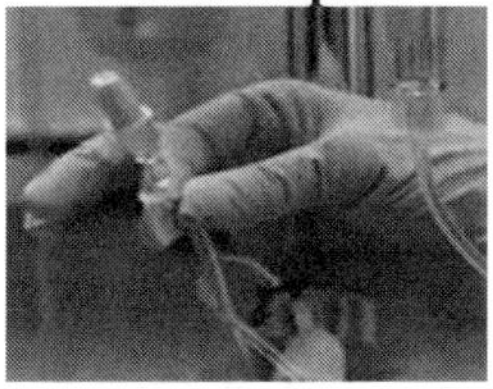

Flush the tubing to drive bubbles along the **line** and safely out.

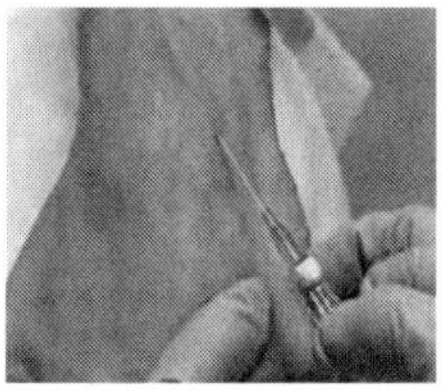

Prep the **skin** with alcohol or Betadine. Insert the **needle** into the **vein**.

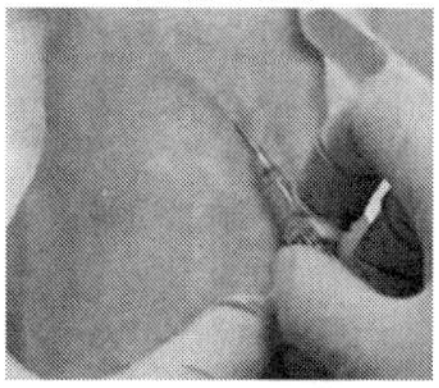

Push the catheter away from the needle with the index finger.

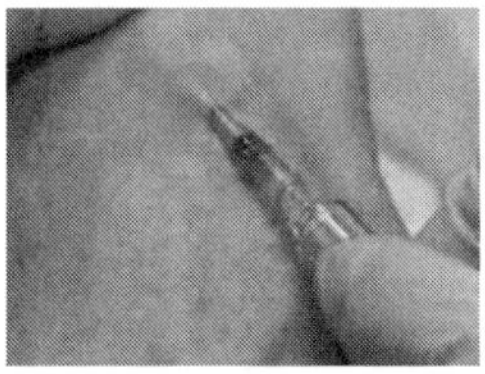

Apply a little pressure to control any **bleed back**.

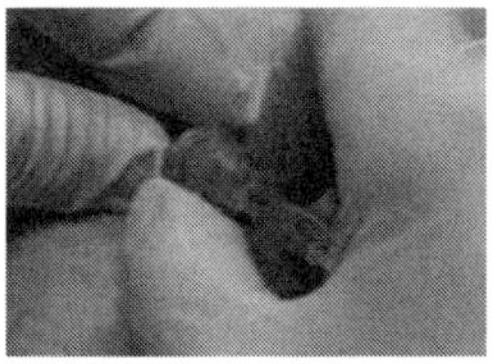

Screw the line firmly into place and check the tubing.

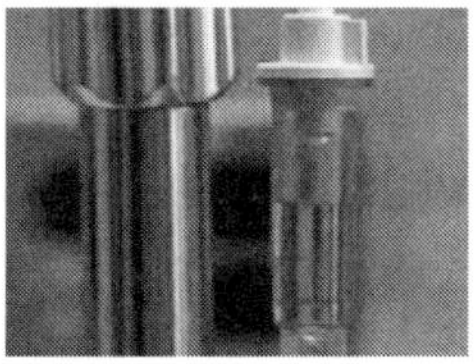

Ensure normal **flow**.

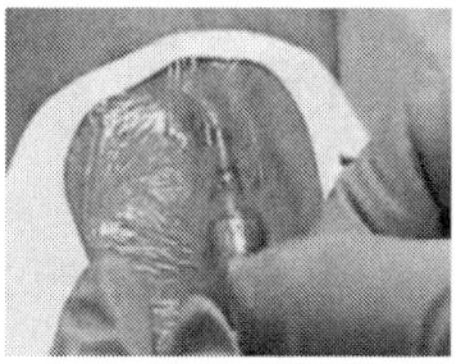

Protect the insertion site.

Word list

(to) hang	pendre / suspendre
tubing	tubulure
spike	perforateur
drip chamber	chambre compte-goutte
full	plein
(to) unroll	dérouler

roller clamp	molette
line	intraveineuse
(to) prep	préparer
skin	peau
needle	aiguille
vein	veine
(to) apply pressure	exercer une pression
bleed back	retour veineux
(to) screw	visser
flow	débit / flux

VIDEO

Blood

http://www.youtube.com/watch?v=CRh_dAzXuoU&feature=related

Script:
What is blood? Blood is actually a mixture of cells suspended in a slightly yellowish liquid called plasma. Plasma is made up mostly of water, but it also contains proteins, sugars, hormones and salts. The three different types of cells you'll find in plasma are red blood cells or erythrocytes, white blood cells or leukocytes, and **platelets** or thrombocytes. Red blood cells give the blood its color and make up 40 to 45% of your blood. But they're round and look a little like a donut without the **hole** in the middle. Their main job is to carry oxygen to the other cells of the body and to **take away** the carbon dioxide as a waste product. Red blood cells only live four months. But healthy **bone marrow** produces four to five billion red cells every hour to keep **replenishing** the ones that **wear out**. White blood cells, on the other hand, are the body's defense system. They all fight infection from bacteria, viruses, all those nasty microbes that can cause disease. Whenever germs begin to infect your body they send out a signal that the granulocyte recognizes. Just as soon as the granulocyte detects the signal, it begins its **journey** to the site of the infection. When at last they finally invade a germ, they quickly move in for the kill, first attacking the invader and then eating it. Something else that is truly amazing is how the platelets work. Platelets are small pieces of solid material or cytoplasm, whose job it is to **plug** holes in the vessel walls. So, say you're standing inside the blood **vessel**, and looking at the **tear** in its wall, you'd see millions of platelets responding to the injury, throwing themselves over the cut. They **stick** to the wound's **edges** and to each other to form a **plug** that slows the **loss** of blood within three to five minutes. A platelet plug will last for only 24 to 72 hours because the platelets **run out of** energy and begin to **fall apart**. But as long as there's still an unhealed hole on the blood vessel wall, the **clot** will continue being formed, dissolved and reformed to stop and prevent more bleeding from occurring. When the wound is completely healed by the new cells **growing over** it, the clot will be **cleared away** and blood will begin to flow through the vessel normally.

Word list

platelet	plaquette
hole	trou
(to) take away	enlever / transporter

bone marrow	moelle osseuse
(to) replenish	remplacer
(to) wear out	s'épuiser
journey	voyage
(to) plug	boucher / obstruer
vessel (blood)	vaisseau (sanguin)
tear	déchirure
(to) stick	se coller
edges (of a wound)	bords / lèvres (d'une plaie)
plug	bouchon
loss	perte
(to) run out of	être à court de
(to) fall apart	se désagréger
clot	caillot
(to) grow over	recouvrir
(to) clear away	dissoudre / éliminer

ADDITIONAL VOCABULARY

arterial blood	sang artériel
venous blood	sang veineux
whole blood	sang entier
full blood count (FBC) (GB) / complete blood count (CBC) (US)	numération formule sanguine (NFS)
red blood cell (RBC)	globule rouge
white blood cell (WBC)	globule blanc
erythrocyte sedimentation rate (ESR)	vitesse de sédimentation (VS)
mean corpuscular volume (MCV)	volume glomérulaire moyen (VGM)
blood electrolytes	ionogramme sanguin
clotting time	temps de coagulation
blood culture	hémoculture

TRANSLATION

1. Written translation: Translate this extract from the video into French.

Their main job is to carry oxygen to the other cells of the body and to take away the carbon dioxide as a waste product. Red blood cells only live four months. But healthy bone marrow produces four to five billion red cells every hour to keep replenishing the ones that wear out. White blood cells on the other hand are the body's defense system. They all fight infection from bacteria, viruses, all those nasty microbes that can cause disease.

2. Translate the following passage into English.

Le sang rentre dans les oreillettes par les veines, puis passe dans les ventricules et ressort par les artères. Les valves cardiaques empêchent le sang de refluer dans le mauvais sens. Chaque battement cardiaque, ou cycle cardiaque, comprend une contraction et relaxation auriculaire, une contraction et relaxation ventriculaire et une courte pause. Un cycle cardiaque normal (au repos) dure 8 dixièmes de seconde. Le sang arrive par la veine cave dans l'oreillette droite. Dans le même temps, le sang oxygéné provenant des poumons arrive par la veine pulmonaire dans l'oreillette gauche. Les muscles des deux oreillettes se contractent et expulsent le sang par les valves auriculo-ventriculaires dans chaque ventricule.

PAIR WORK

1. Translate this extract as an oral pair work activity.
Student 1 translates the passage below into French, section by section.
Student 2 listens to the translation and translates back into English.
Student 1 listens to the new English version and asks **student 2** to make changes when necessary.

Platelets are small pieces of solid material or cytoplasm, whose job it is to plug holes in the vessel walls. So, say you're standing inside the blood vessel, and looking at the tear in its wall, you'd see millions of platelets responding to the injury, throwing themselves over the cut. They stick to the wound's edges and to each other to form a plug that slows the loss of blood within three to five minutes.

2. Using the pictures at the end of the book (**File 3**, p. 161)**, student 1** explains to **student 2** how to set up an I.V.

Chapter 17

INSULIN INJECTIONS / PIQÛRES D'INSULINE

NURSING SKILLS: SELF-ADMINISTERED INJECTIONS

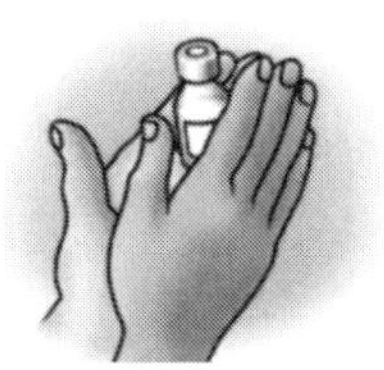

Roll **vial** gently between hands.

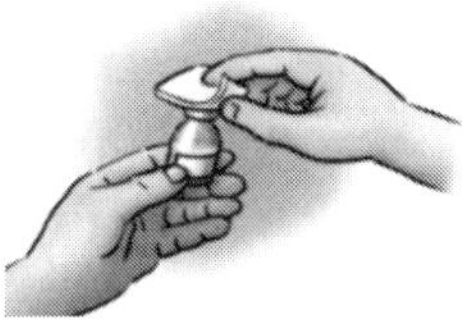

Wipe top of vial with **alcohol swab.**

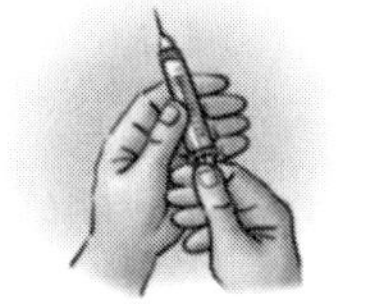

Remove needle cap.

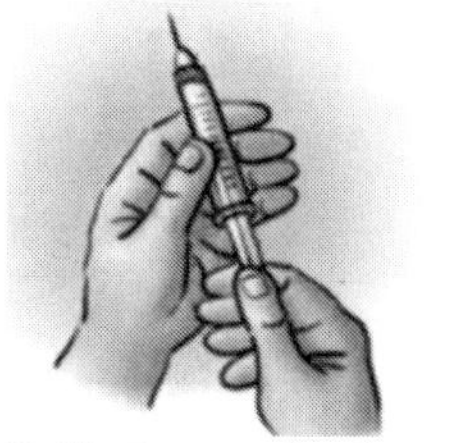

Pull **plunger** back to your dose.

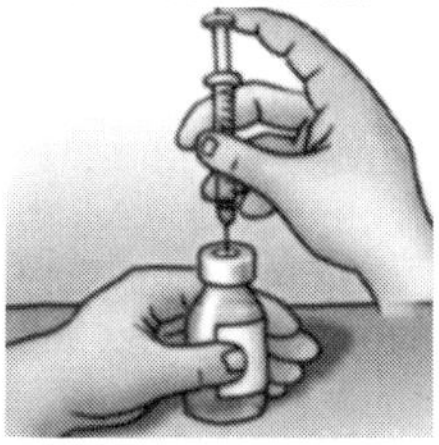

Insert needle into vial and push plunger down.

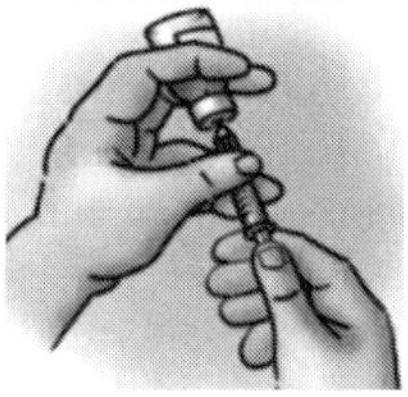

Turn vial **upside down** and pull plunger back to your dose.

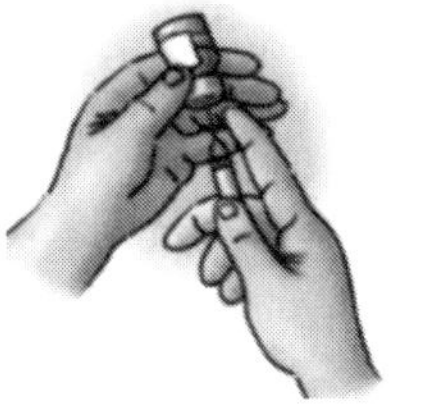

Remove syringe and needle from vial.

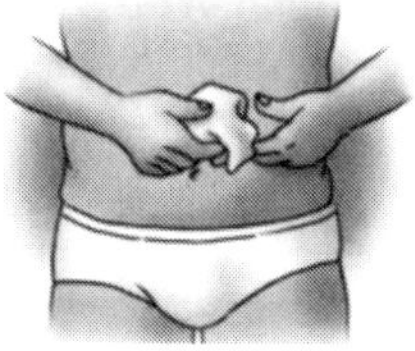

Wipe skin of **chosen** site with alcohol.

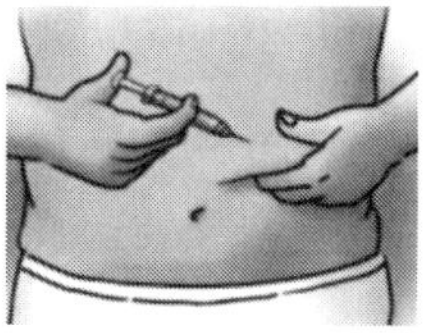

Pinch skin and insert needle at 80 - 90°.

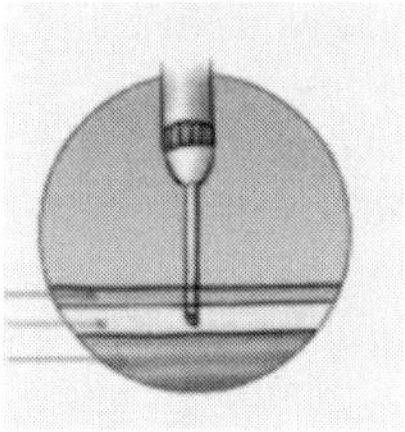

Inject insulin into subcutaneous tissue.

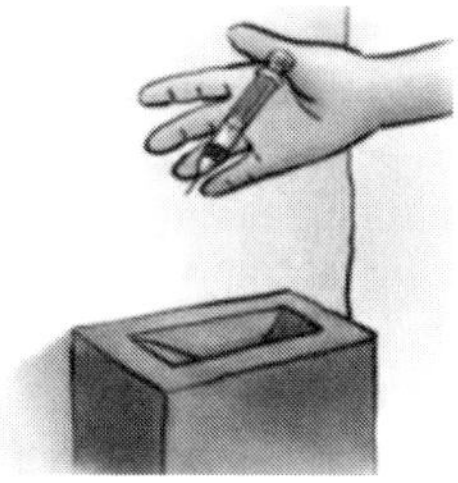

Discard syringe and needle.

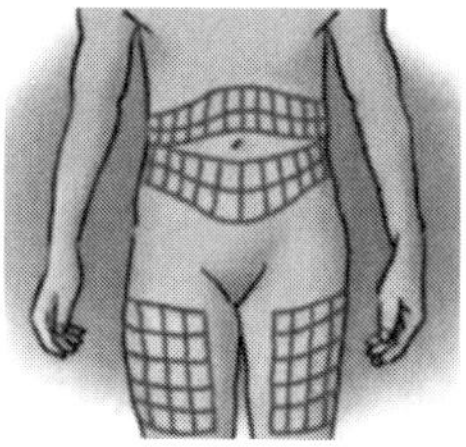

Change injection site regularly.

Word list

vial	ampoule / fiole
(alcohol) swab	tampon (d'alcool)
plunger	piston
upside down	à l'envers
chosen	choisi
(to) discard	jeter

VIDEO

Islet injection for diabetics

http://www.youtube.com/watch?v=wgYMerixS4Q

Script:

Journalist: Kimberley and her two daughters take four insulin injections a day. A **drop in blood sugar** while they sleep could **prove** fatal, so Kimberley has to get up during the night to check everyone's **glucose levels**.
Kimberley Hall: If I don't have my husband, I have to have someone else with me during the night cos' sometimes I can have really bad low blood sugars during the night, which I don't feel, no I don't feel it at all, and that's why I always have to have someone with me.
Journalist: Three years ago, Kimberley had a pancreas transplant and thought her days of insulin jabs were **over**, but last November her body rejected the organ. Another transplant would be very risky, but in this **lab** they're creating an alternative. Scottish **medics** are developing a technique which extracts the insulin-producing cells from a pancreas. The cells, called **islets**, can then be injected into a patient under anaesthetic. For Type I diabetes **sufferers**, it could one day become a **cure**.
Doctor John Casey: Clearly, at present, there will be a minority of patients who will be insulin independent, but I think this is the first **step** in a... in a programme for Scottish patients. I, you know, I would hope that... that, that we aren't looking too far in the future to really **achieve** stem cell transplantation for diabetes.
Journalist: How would it be for you one day if you didn't have to take injections?
Amy Hall: Good. It would be amazing to think that I would get up in the morning just not thinking about, like, having jabs and blood tests.
Journalist: Initially, only twelve patients a year will be able to receive the islet treatment, but for the 30,000 Type I diabetes sufferers across Scotland, like Kimberley and her girls, the work **going on** in this lab offers the hope of not only an **injection-free** life but a full night's sleep.

Word list

drop in	chute de
blood sugar	glycémie
(to) prove (fatal)	s'avérer (fatal)
glucose level	taux de glycémie

over	terminé
lab(oratoty)	labo(ratoire)
medic	médecin
islet	îlot
sufferer	malade
cure	guérison
step	étape
(to)achieve	réaliser/ accomplir
going on	en cours
injection-free	sans piqûre

ADDITIONAL VOCABULARY

injection / shot / jab	injection / piqûre
intravenous (IV)	intraveineux (IV)
intramuscular (IM)	intramusculaire (IM)
subcutaneous (SC)	sous-cutané (SC)
inoculation	inoculation
disposable	jetable
needle disposal container	boîte jette-aiguilles
needle-stick injury	blessure par piqûre d'aiguille
(to) stick in the needle	planter l'aiguille
barrel (of the syringe)	corps (de la seringue)
sharp end	extrémité pointue
(to) disinfect	désinfecter
insulin pen	stylo à insuline

TRANSLATION

1. Translate the following sentences into English.

1. Avez-vous fait vérifier votre taux de glycémie récemment ?
2. La plupart des patients, qui ont un diabète de type I, s'habituent rapidement aux piqûres d'insuline.
3. Il est stupéfiant de penser que si peu de malades bénéficient de ce traitement.
4. Avez-vous entendu parler de la recherche sur les cellules souche ?
5. C'est la première étape du nouveau programme de vaccination lancé par le gouvernement.

2. Written translation: Translate this abstract into French.

Introduction

The goal of this study was to evaluate the effectiveness on post-operative pain and the impact on cognitive function, of patient-controlled analgesia (PCA) compared with subcutaneous (SC) injections of morphine in elderly patients undergoing total hip replacement (THR).

Methods

Forty patients older than 70 years were randomly assigned to two different postoperative analgesic techniques for 48 hours: IV PCA morphine dose 1 mg (PCA group) or regular SC morphine injections (SC group). Postoperative pain was assessed at rest and when moving using a visual analogue scale (VAS) every 4 h. A Mini Mental Status Examination (MMSE) was used to assess cognitive function before surgery, at 2 h, 24 h and 48 h after surgery and at hospital discharge. Side-effects were also recorded during the first 24 h after surgery.

Results

The PCA group showed significantly lower pain scores than the SC group both at rest and during mobilization. There was no intergroup difference in post-operative MMS scores. The incidence of side-effects was similar in both groups.

Conclusions

We conclude that in healthy elderly subjects undergoing THR, the flexibility of the analgesic regimen is more important than the route of administration with regard to efficacy, adverse effects and recovery of cognitive function.

Key words: elderly; analgesia; patient-controlled; morphine; pain; post-operative surgery; total hip replacement.

PAIR WORK

Using the pictures at the end of the book (**File 4**, p. 162)**, student 1** explains to **student 2** how to give an injection.

Chapter 18

DRESSING A WOUND / PANSER UNE PLAIE

NURSING SKILLS: CHANGING A DRESSING

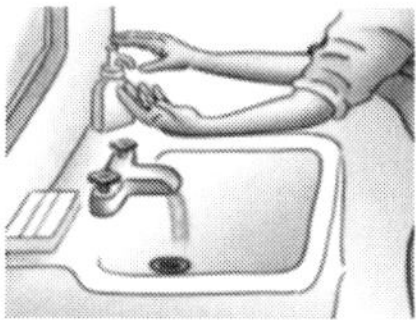
Carefully wash and **dry** your hands.

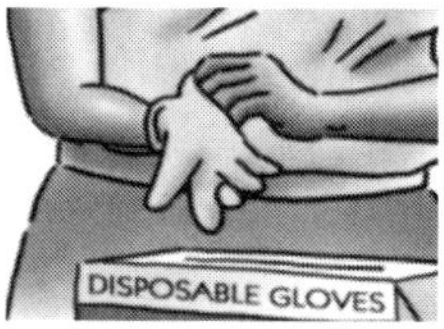

Put on your gloves.

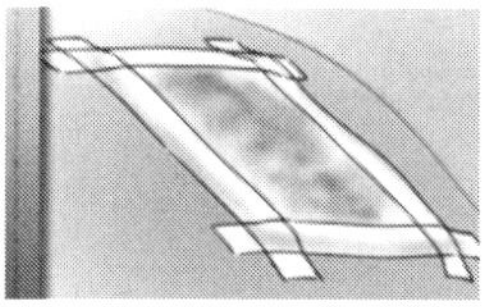
Remove the old dressing.

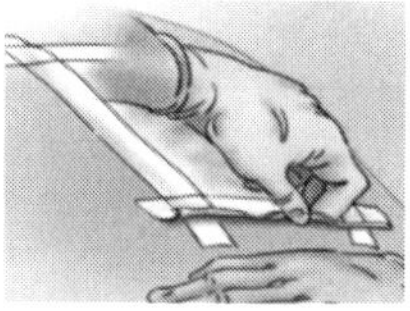
Unstick the edges of the **tape** keeping the skin **taut** by the other hand.

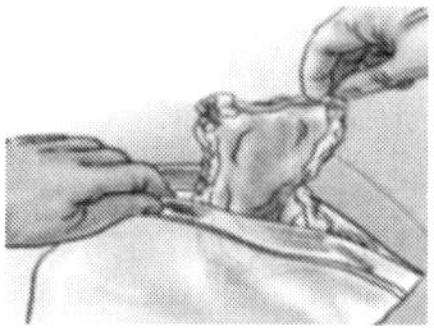
Dispose of the old dressing.

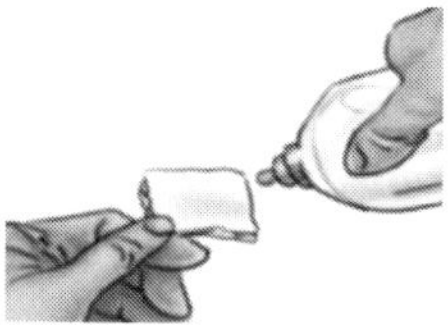
Pour some **cleansing solution** onto a gauze **pad**.

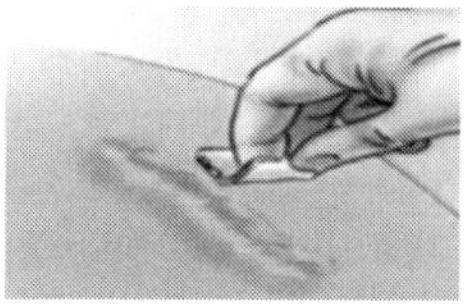
Clean the wound from top to bottom.

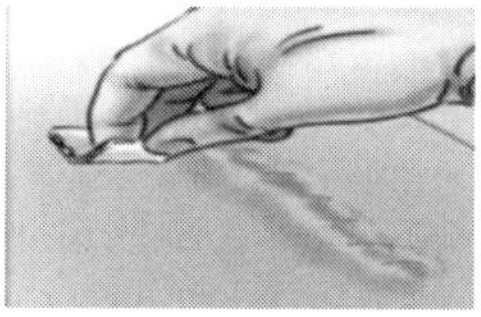
Clean the skin for about 7 centimeters from the wound on either side.

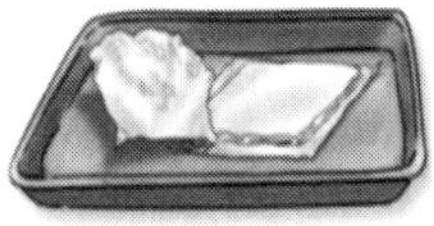
Open a package of large gauze dressing.

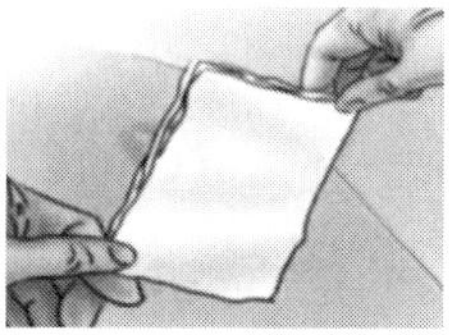
Pick up the dressing gauze by opposite corners, center the pad and place it over the wound.

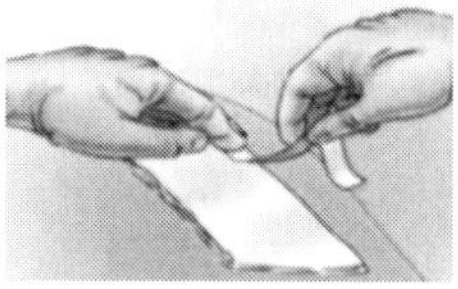
Fix the dressing securely in place with tape.

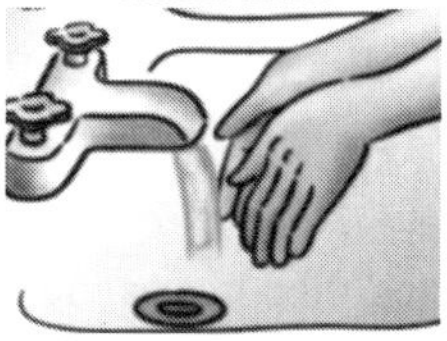
Dispose of the used gloves, and wash and dry your hands.

Word list

(to) dry	*sécher*
(to) unstick	*décoller*
tape	*sparadrap*
taut	*étiré / tendu*
cleansing solution	*solution de rinçage (de plaie)*
pad	*tampon / compresse*
(to) pick up	*se saisir de*

VIDEO

Sterile Dressing sutured wound

http://www.youtube.com/watch?v=vvDxQgH9x-8

Script:
Now let's **go ahead** and demonstrate **applying** a dry sterile dressing to an adult client's surgical wound. We'll assume the nurse has checked the **provider's** orders, **screened** the client **for** allergies and explained the procedure to the client. The nurse assembles her equipment. She will need a towel or **waterproof pad**, a **bath blanket**, clean gloves, a **moisture-proof biohazard bag**, **adhesive remover**, a sterile dressing kit or the appropriate dressing materials, sterile **drapes** and the prescribed cleansing solution, tape, **straps** or a **binder**, sterile gloves and any other materials the provider specifies, such as ointment. Next, the nurse provides privacy and assists the client into a comfortable position that allows good access to the **surgical** wound. She protects the **bed linen** with a towel or pad. With the bath blanket, she covers the client appropriately, except for the area where the dressing is. She sets up the **disposal bag** for easy access, then washes her hands and puts on clean gloves. Gently, she removes the existing dressing. Applying counter traction to the skin, she **peels** the tape **away**, all the while being careful not to pull on the sutures or on any drains. If the adhesive were to resist removal, she would use a solvent to **loosen** the tape. She places the removed dressing in the disposal bag without touching the outside of the bag and noting the characteristics of any **drainage** on the dressing. She then removes the clean gloves and washes hers hands. Next, she assesses the wound so that she can later **document** her **findings**. She opens all sterile supplies and **pours** the cleansing solution into a sterile basin. She puts on her sterile gloves and carefully **cleanses** the wound following the provider's orders or the institution's policy. Note that she cleanses it from the area of least contamination to the area of most contamination, using one sterile swab, gauze or cotton ball for each **stroke**. If this wound had a drain, she would cleanse it and the surrounding skin last. She dries the area completely with gauze pads. If any medication has been prescribed, she would apply it. If this wound had a drain, she would apply pre-cut gauze around it, extra gauze below it, and **add** dressing material over it to collect drainage. Next, the nurse applies the sterile dressing over the wound. For larger wounds, the final covering is usually an abdominal pad to absorb drainage and protect it from trauma.

Finally, she **secures** the dressing with tape or straps. If the client has fragile or sensitive skin, she'd be sure to use paper tape. After changing any dressing, you remove your glove and dispose of them in the proper receptacle. Make sure the client is comfortable, then wash your hands. Document your dressing change, your assessment of the wound, any drainage or **fluids** on the dressing you removed, and their color and odor, any wound care you provided, how the client tolerated the procedure, and any other concerns or observations in the client's **record**. Some institution or protocols also require that you put the date, the time and your initials on the new dressing, so that there is no question about when the dressing was last changed.

Word list

(to)go ahead	continuer / reprendre
(to) apply	faire (un pansement) / appliquer
provider	médecin soignant
(to) screen (for)	dépister / repérer
waterproof pad	champ de soins (imperméable)
bath blanket	alèse / serviette
moisture proof	étanche
biohazard bag	sac biohazard
adhesive remover	dissolvant à colle
drapes	champ stérile
strap	bande
binder	bandage abdominal
surgical	chirurgical
bed linen	literie
disposal bag	sac à déchets
(to) peel away	décoller / retirer
(to) loosen	(ici) ramollir
drainage	écoulement
(to) document	noter / enregistrer
finding	résultat
(to) cleanse	nettoyer
(to) pour	verser
stroke	passage / application
(to) add	ajouter
(to) secure	fixer
fluids	liquides
record	dossier

ADDITIONAL VOCABULARY

pus	pus
(to) ooze	suinter / suppurer
scab / crust	croûte
scar / scarring	cicatrice
wound healing	cicatrisation

infection	infection
(to) become infected	s'infecter
debridement	débridement / mise à plat
swollen	gonflé / boursoufflé
purulent / suppurating	purulent
malodorous / stinky / foul-smelling	malodorant / puant / nauséabond
bedsore	escarre
butterfly stitches	steri-strip®

TRANSLATION

1. Written translation: Translate this extract from the video into French.
Gently, she removes the existing dressing. Applying counter traction to the skin, she peels the tape away all the while being careful not to pull on the sutures or on any drains. If the adhesive were to resist removal, she would use a solvent to loosen the tape. She places the removed dressing in the disposal bag without touching the outside of the bag and noting the characteristics of any drainage on the dressing. She then removes the clean gloves and washes hers hands. Next, she assesses the wound so that she can later document her findings.

2. Written translation: Translate the following passage into French.
Suturing is closing a wound surgically, using stitches or staples. Proper cleansing in care of sutured wounds will promote faster healing with better approximation of the wound's edges and will reduce the risk of complications. Proper application of the sterile dressing protects the wound from trauma, reduces the risk of bacterial infection and promotes healing.

PAIR WORK

Using the pictures at the end of the book **(File 5**, p. 162)**, student 1** explains to **student 2** how to change a dressing.

Chapter 19

BLOOD PRESSURE AND HEART DISEASE / LA TENSION ARTERIELLE ET LES MALADIES CARDIAQUES

NURSING SKILLS: TAKING A PATIENT'S BLOOD PRESSURE

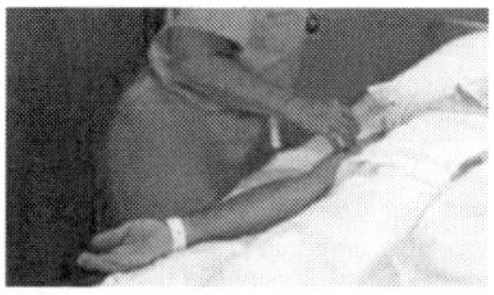

Expose the upper arm fully by removing any **clothing** that is **in the way**.

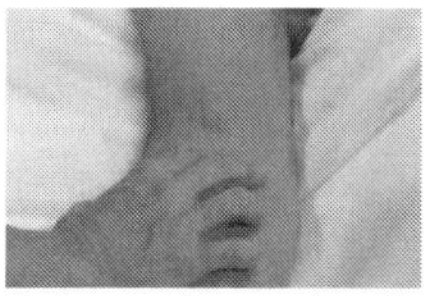

Palpate the patient's brachial artery.

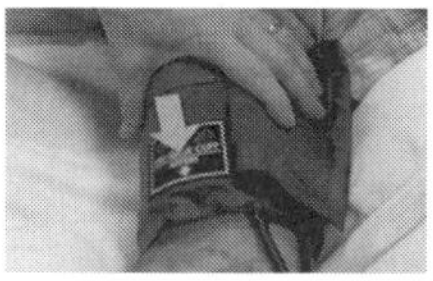

Position the **cuff** over the artery. **Wrap** the fully **deflated** cuff around the upper arm.

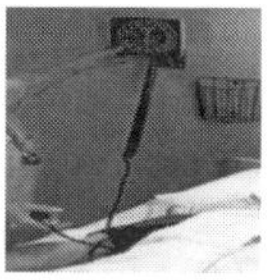

Position the manometer vertically at eye level.

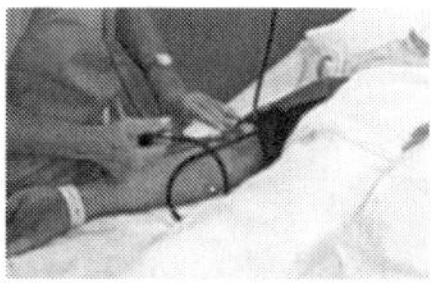

Place the **stethoscope bell** or **diaphragm** over the artery.

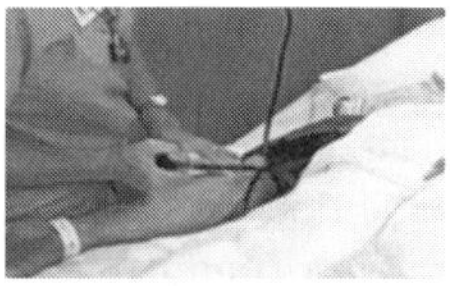

Palpate the brachial artery while **inflating** the cuff.

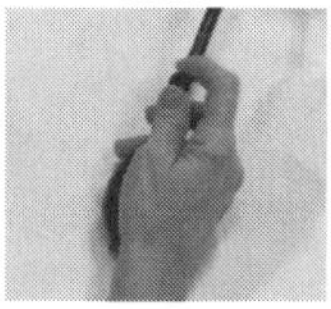

Close the valve on the **pressure bulb**. Quickly inflate the cuff.

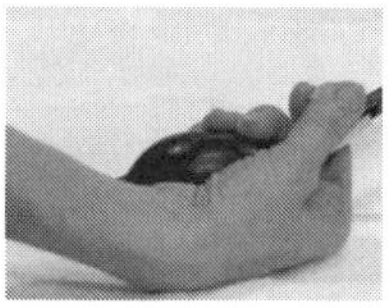

Slowly **release** the valve on the pressure bulb.

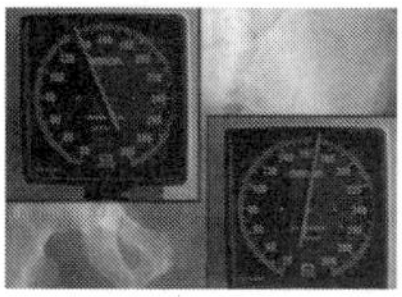

Note the point when you hear the first clear sound. This is the systolic pressure.

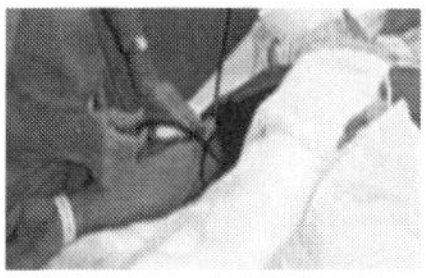

When the sound disappears, note the pressure which **deflects** the diastolic pressure needle.

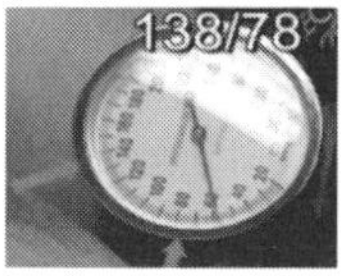

Let the remaining air **escape** quickly: one (hundred and) thirty-eight over seventy-eight.

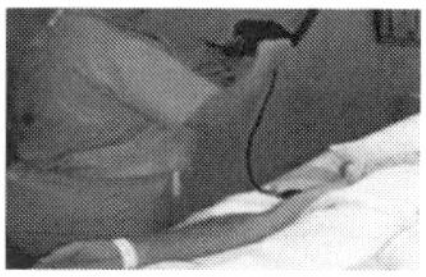

Remove the cuff from the patient's arm.

Word list

clothing	vêtement
(to be) in the way	gêner
cuff	brassard
(to) wrap	enrouler
(to) deflate	dégonfler
stethoscope bell	pavillon
stethoscope diaphragm	membrane
(to) inflate	gonfler
(pressure) bulb	poire
(to) release	dévisser / ouvrir
(to) deflect	dévier / infléchir
(to) escape	s'échapper

VIDEO

Nurses fight heart disease

http://www.youtube.com/watch?v=mECt79rOa90

Script:
Journalist: It's the number one killer of men and women in the United States today. It **strikes** every thirty-seven seconds and is responsible for more than two thousand American deaths each day. Heart disease is known as the silent killer and medical experts say it's crucial to be educated about personal **risk factors** for heart attack and stroke.
Kathy Berra: There are a number of personal risk factors that put us at risk for heart attack and stroke. These include cigarette smoking, **high blood pressure**, elevated cholesterol, type II diabetes. Other things like being physically inactive, **weighing** too much, eating not a **heart-healthy diet** and personal stress can all put us at risk. If you have a male in your family under the age of 55 or a woman under the age of 65 with heart disease, you're also at **increased** risk. When you combine any of these risk factors like diabetes and being **overweight** and having high blood pressure, again your risk becomes even higher.
Journalist: Healthcare providers **agree** that **awareness** is the **key** to prevention and early detection of heart disease and stroke. For the past 15 years, the Preventive Cardiovascular Nurses Association has been committed to educating and **promoting** the important role of nurses in the prevention and treatment of this national **epidemic**. PCNA takes a **hands-on approach** by engaging patients to identify personal risk factors, helping them to **implement lifestyle** and **behavioral** changes and **seek** the proper medical therapies. PCNA believes these combined strategies can reduce their risk for heart disease and stroke.
Nancy Houston Miller: Preventive Cardiovascular Nurses Association was really developed by nurses to **train** nurses to prevent and **manage** cholesterol. Over the past 15 years, we've dealt with all cardiovascular risk factors and we reach one million individuals annually. PCNA is really committed to working with individuals across the **lifespan**. For example, we **advocate for** better nutrition in schools to prevent overweight and obesity,

increasing physical activity in schools and for the older adults, we recommend high blood pressure monitoring in order to increase blood pressure control.
Journalist: Statistics show that nearly one fourth of Americans have some form of heart disease. Through prevention and education strategies, PCNA is committed to helping Americans protect their hearts and live healthier, longer lives.

Word list

(to) strike	frapper
risk factor	facteur de risque
high blood pressure (HBP)	hypertension artérielle
(to) weigh	peser
heart-healthy diet	régime alimentaire sain pour le cœur
(to) increase	augmenter
overweight	surpoids / en surpoids
(to) agree	être d'accord
awareness	conscience
key	(élément) clef
(to) promote	promouvoir
epidemic	épidémie
hands-on approach	approche pragmatique
(to) implement	mettre en œuvre
lifestyle	mode de vie / règles hygiéno-diététiques
behavioral	comportemental
(to) seek	(re)chercher
(to) train	former
(to) manage	prendre en charge
lifespan	durée de vie
(to) advocate (for)	préconiser

ADDITIONAL VOCABULARY

angina	angine de poitrine / angor
aortic dissection	dissection aortique
arrhythmia	arythmie
atherosclerosis	athérosclérose
atrial fibrillation	fibrillation auriculaire
AV block	bloc auriculo-ventriculaire
bradycardia	bradycardie
cardiac arrest	arrêt cardiaque
coronary artery bypass graft (CABG)	pontage coronarien
coronary artery disease	maladie coronarienne
heart failure	insuffisance cardiaque
myocardial infarction (MI)/heart attack	infarctus du myocarde / crise cardiaque
pericarditis	péricardite
tachycardia	tachycardie
valvular heart disease	valvulopathie / cardiopathie valvulaire
ventricular fibrillation	fibrillation ventriculaire

TRANSLATION

1. Translate the following sentences into English.

1. De nos jours, le surpoids peut être considéré comme une épidémie mondiale.
2. Le chocolat est peut-être bon pour le cœur, mais il est souvent interdit en cas de diabète.
3. Cette brochure explique comment une crise cardiaque ou une attaque cérébrale survient et comment on peut l'éviter.
4. Ce stage va former les infirmières à reconnaître tous les signes de l'hypertension.
5. De nombreuses maladies cardiaques frappent à partir de 50 ans.

2. Written translation: Translate the following passage into French.

There is no BP value above which you must always treat and below which you can safely ignore. You must always take into account family history, age, smoking and lipid status - and more complex matters such as the value a patient sets on life. If the patient agrees, involve the spouse or partner in the decision to implement treatment. No one remembers to take antihypertensive medication all the time, and the spouse may be more motivated to get the treatment right if the patient does not think life is worth living. It may be useful to spend time treating the patient's depression before talking about antihypertensives.

In 95% of cases the cause of hypertension is unknown, though alcohol consumption and overweight may play a role. This is called essential hypertension. A variety of diseases can be at the root of hypertension in the other 5% of cases.

Presentations include headache, stroke, heart failure, MI, kidney failure, and even blindness.

PAIR WORK

Using the pictures at the end of the book (**File 6,** p. 163), **student 1** explains to **student 2** how to take a patient's blood pressure.

Chapter 20

PREVENTION OF NOSOCOMIAL INFECTIONS / LA PREVENTION DES MALADIES NOSOCOMIALES

NURSING SKILLS: HAND-WASHING

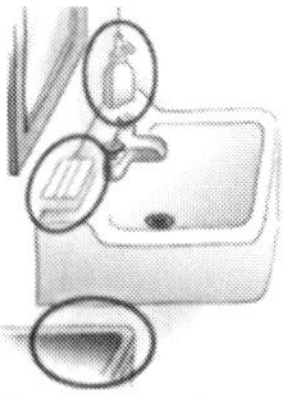

Make sure there is a **soap dispenser**, paper towel and a **bin nearby**.

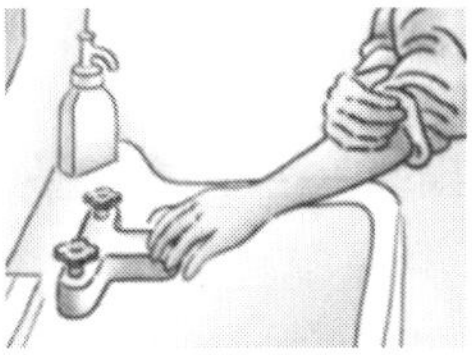

Push your **sleeves** up away from your hands.

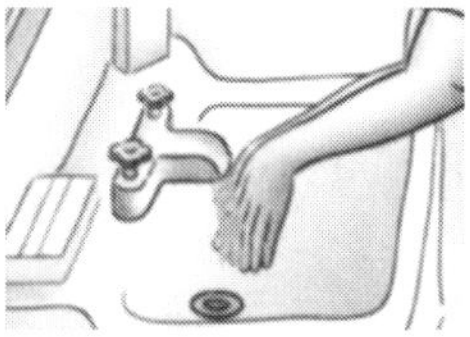

Point your fingers down and **wet** your hands with **warm** water.

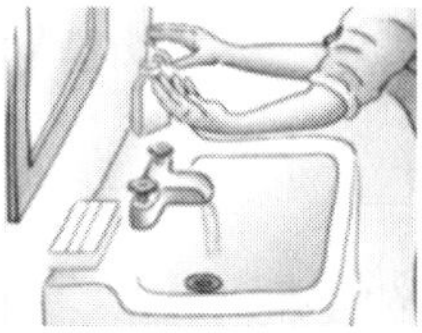

Apply soap from the dispenser.

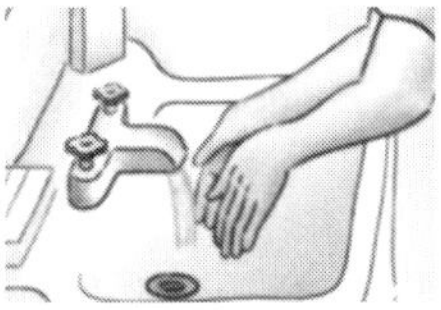

Rub your hands vigorously together in a circular motion.

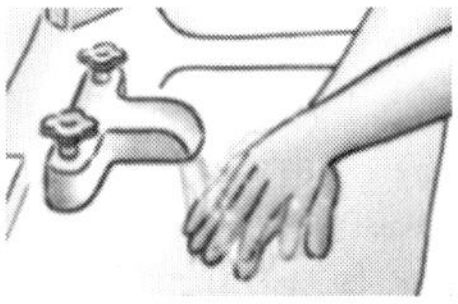

Intertwine your fingers to clean all parts of your hands.

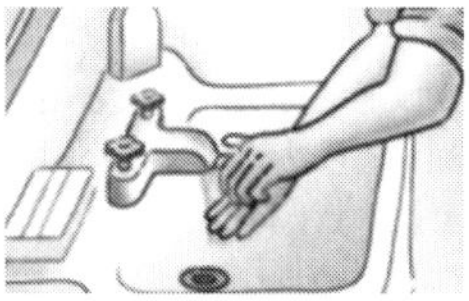

Rub your **fingernails** in the **palm** of your other hand.

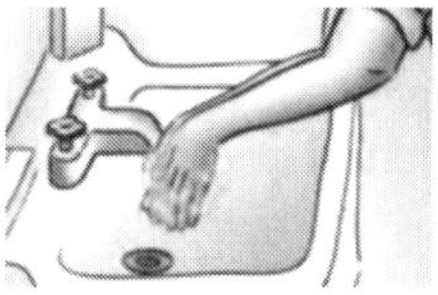

Rinse your hands from the wrist to **fingertips**.

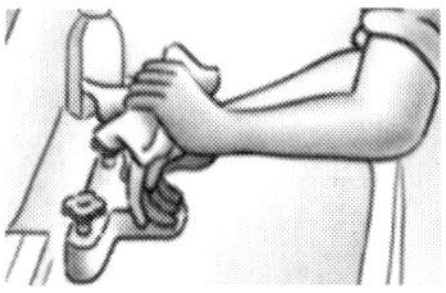

Carefully dry your hands with a clean paper towel.

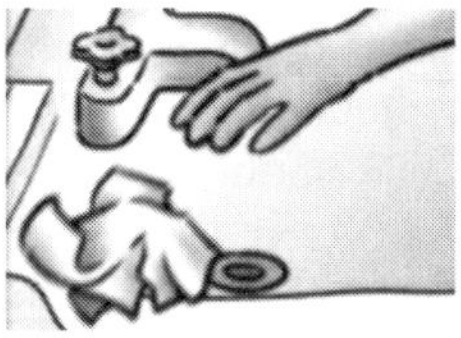

Discard the paper towel into the bin.

Word list

(to) make sure	vérifier / s'assurer que
soap dispenser	distributeur de savon
bin	poubelle

nearby	à proximité
sleeve	manche
(to) wet	mouiller
warm	chaud
(to) rub	frotter
(to) intertwine	(entre)croiser
(finger)nail	ongle
palm	paume
fingertip	extrémité du doigt

VIDEO

MRSA

http://www.youtube.com/watch?v=47KBVPhY4Zs

Script:
Journalist: The **fight** against **MRSA** is **relentless**. Here in Harrogate, specialist teams called ward hygienists have just been introduced to **target** equipment that's constantly moved around wards such as blood pressure monitors.
Fiona Boland: Do you mind doing some hand hygiene, Jill?
Hand hygiene champions encourage all visitors and staff in Harrogate to wash their hands and be vigilant about hygiene, and it seems to be working.
Fiona Boland: **Mostly**, everyone's been really positive and I think, as the months have gone on, people have become a lot more aware of, like, how important it is and people are like, a lot more **responsive** to do it.
Journalist: Every **hospital trust** has been introducing new measures to prevent MRSA, and according to today's **figures,** it's working. In England, in June 2006, there were 1,742 reported cases of MRSA **bloodstream infections**. In June 2007, that had reduced to just over 1,300 cases. And now for June 2008, the figure is even lower, at 836. In the hospital labs, they're constantly checking for new cases.
Kevin Kerr: So what we've got here is MRSA **growing** on a **culture dish**; we have little paper discs which contain different types of antibiotics. If the MRSA is killed by an antibiotic, it can't grow around the disc and you see it's nice and clear here. If, however, the MRSA is resistant to the antibiotic, it grows right up to the disc.
Journalist: Professor Kevin Kerr says while people associate MRSA with hospitals, patients often bring in the infection on admission, and certain groups are at higher risk.
Kevin Kerr: From our **data**, we know that these are older patients who are being admitted to the hospital as emergencies; they're the patients who we find are most **likely to** get MRSA, that's why we screen them.
No fun to have MRSA…
Journalist: This hospital's radio station even has its own song **warning** of the dangers of **superbugs**. At the **frontline**, hospitals need plenty of **weapons** to fight these infections.

Word list

fight	combat
MRSA (methicillin-resistant staphylococcus aureus)	SARM (staphylococcus aureus résistant à la méthicilline)
relentless	acharné / sans merci
(to) target	cibler
mostly	la plupart du temps
responsive	réactif / sensible à
hospital trust (GB)	hôpital public (autonome)
figure	chiffre
bloodstream	circulation sanguine
bloodstream infection	bactériémie
(to) grow	se développer / proliférer
culture dish	boîte de culture
data (pl)	données
likely to	susceptible de
(to) warn	avertir
superbug	bactérie multi-résistante (BMR)
frontline	première ligne / front
weapon	arme

ADDITIONAL VOCABULARY

bug / germ	germe / microbe
alcohol-based hand-rubs	gel hydro alcoolique pour les mains
strain	souche
airborne infection	infection d'origine aérienne
foodborne infection	infection d'origine alimentaire
waterborne infection	infection d'origine hydrique
hospital-acquired infection	infection hospitalière
community-acquired infection	infection communautaire
fungus (pl fungi)	champignon
fungal infection	mycose
legionnaire's disease	maladie du légionnaire
legionellosis	légionellose
(to) pass on (an infection)	transmettre (une infection)
(to) spread to	se transmettre à
(to) sneeze	éternuer
(to) cough	tousser
bleach	eau de javel
chlorine	chlore
ammonia	ammoniaque

TRANSLATION

1. Translate the following sentences into English.

1. Les hygiénistes hospitaliers jouent un rôle clef dans la prévention d'infections nosocomiales qui sont souvent introduites par les patients.
2. Les bactériémies dues au SARM chez des patients hospitalisés dans des services chirurgicaux sont souvent très graves.
3. Il est important d'examiner soigneusement les patients, le jour même de leur admission à l'hôpital, afin de détecter toute présence de microbes pathogènes.
4. Tout le personnel de l'hôpital est en première ligne pour combattre les bactéries multi-résistantes.

2. Written translation: Translate the following passage into French.

Person-to-person contact and contaminated surfaces are the cause of large outbreaks of viral gastroenteritis. These observations underlined the need for good hygiene standards to prevent nosocomial outbreaks in clinical institutions (e.g. hospitals, nursing homes). In this study, we evaluated surface disinfectants (bleach, ammonia solutions) and hand-cleaning products (alcohol-based hand-rubs, betadine), which are routinely used in hospitals. It is interesting to note that the disinfectants we tested were primarily selected by the hospital because they are well tolerated by the users (e.g. healthcare professionals and patients), and for their efficacy against microbial pathogens and viruses.

Chlorine-based disinfectants such as bleach are cheap and among the most effective virucidal disinfectants available. Previous studies showed that 1,000 to 3,000 ppm of chlorine were enough to inactivate many strains of pathogenic viruses.

PAIR WORK

Using the pictures at the end of the book (**File 7**, p. 163), **student 1** explains to **student 2** how to wash one's hands.

Chapter 21

BLOOD DONATION AND BLOOD TRANSFUSION / DON DU SANG ET TRANSFUSION SANGUINE

NURSING SKILLS: TAKING A BLOOD SAMPLE

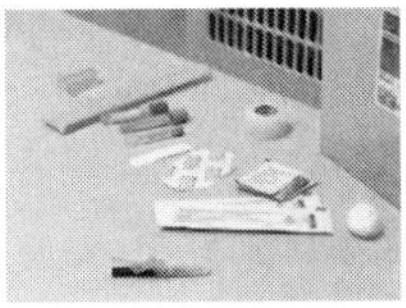

Wash your hands carefully, put on sterile gloves and get your **blood tubes** and needle ready.

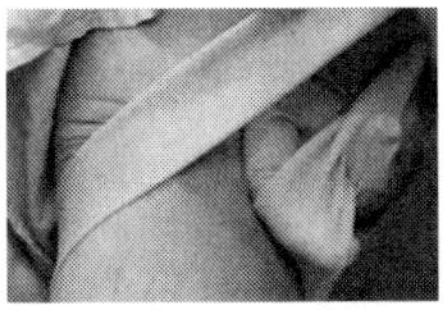

Place the **tourniquet flat** on the patient's arm. Pull on each end and form an X.

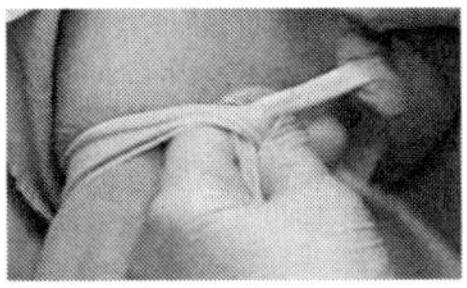

Bring the front **tail** around the X and form a **loop** pointing downward.

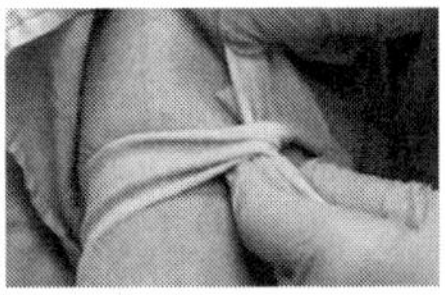

Remove your finger and leave the tails hanging.

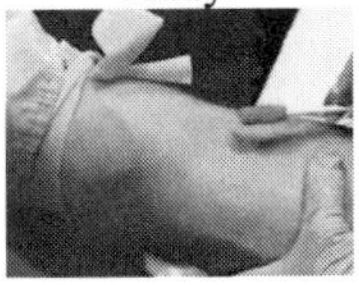

Carefully cleanse the skin with alcohol.

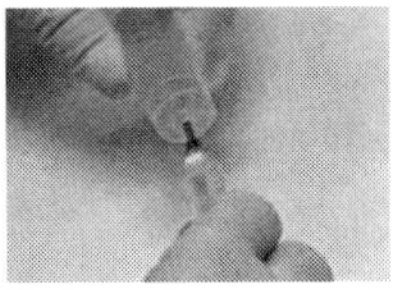

Carefully remove the cap to **unsheathe** the needle. Insert it into the vacutainer and screw it into place.

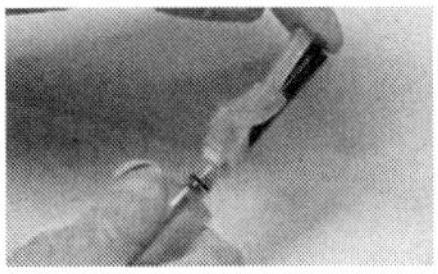

Lift the **needle guard**.

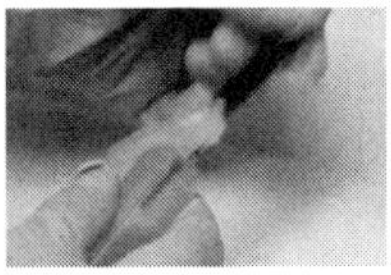

Remove the cap.

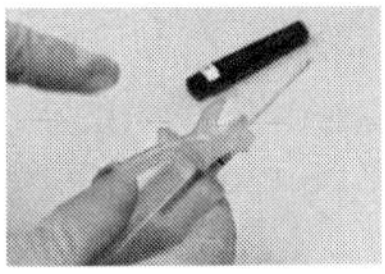

The hole in the edge of the needle is facing up.

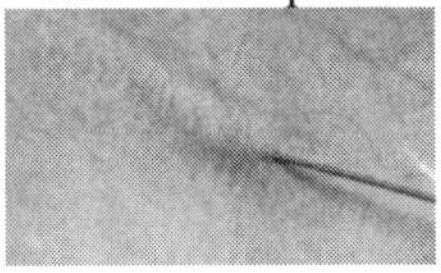

Approach the vein at a **shallow angle**.

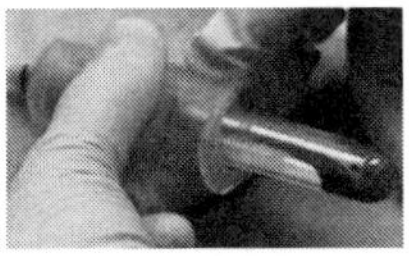

The blood flows back into the vacutainer.

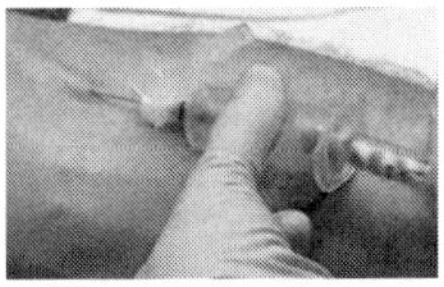

To **switch** tubes, **steady** your hand against the arm.

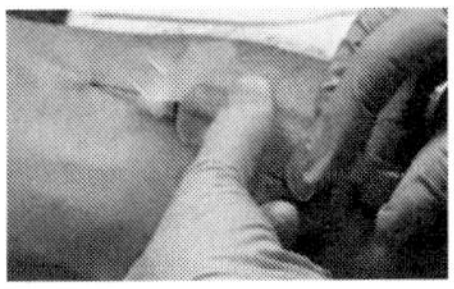

Insert the next tube without pushing the needle any deeper.

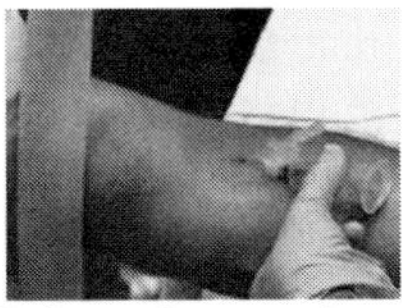

Release the tourniquet by pulling on one or both tails.

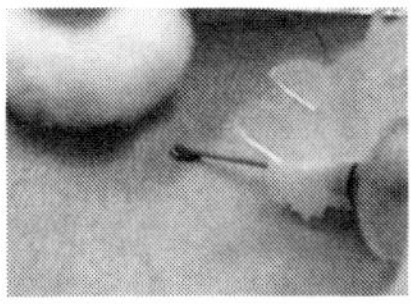

Place the cotton ball above the **puncture** site.

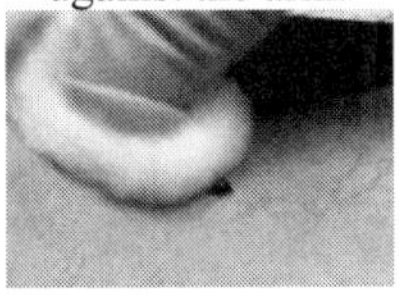

Withdraw the needle straight back.

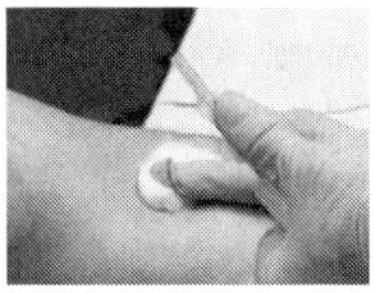

Roll the cotton gently over the puncture site and apply a steady pressure.

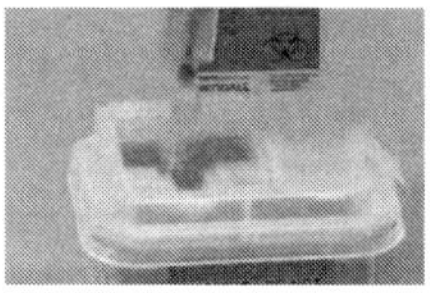

Discard the needle into the container.

Word list

blood tube	tube (de prélèvement)
tourniquet	garrot
flat	(à) plat
tail	extrémité du lien
loop	boucle
(to) unsheathe	retirer de sa gaine de protection
needle guard	gaine de protection
shallow angle	angle relativement faible
(to) switch	changer de
(to) steady one's hand	garder la main ferme
puncture	ponction
(to) withdraw	retirer

VIDEO

Synthetic blood

http://www.youtube.com/watch?v=XDxZlmy8l3Y

Script:

Sir Richard Branson: Without this woman, my father couldn't have had his hip replaced.

Sue Saville: Celebrities have **lent** their voices to the **plea** for more blood donors. It's a constant effort to renew fresh blood supplies, but now British **scientists** believe they can produce red blood cells of the rare but universally tolerated O-negative blood group by using stem cells from human embryos.

Pr Mark Turner: Over the next three years, what we would like to do is achieve **proof of principle** that we can indeed produce red cells of the kind of **grade** that **behave** rather like a red cell transfusion a patient would receive today. And then after that, of course, there will be a challenge in terms of **scaling up** that technology to produce the kinds and numbers of red blood cells that we would require for routine transfusions.

Saville: Blood donations have become an essential part of health care. Last year in England, 1.6 million people gave blood, which **sounds** a lot but that's just 4% of the **eligible** population. Eight thousand units are needed each day, but the blood must be used within a month.

Journalist: Each of these units of blood has been given by a **willing** volunteer, but there's **concern** that creating synthetic blood using stem cells from human embryos discarded after **IVF** treatment could **raise** serious ethical issues.

Experts hope this could be **overcome** by needing only small numbers of embryos to start this **self-renewing** process.
Pr John Gribben: It's been the **Holy Grail** of medicine to try to find ways to be able to replenish blood. To create this synthetically means that, not only do we have no limit to the supply of the blood, but we have a supply of the blood free of the risk of any potential transmission of infectious agents.
Saville: In theory, one day blood donors won't be needed, but the **leap** to mass blood production is at least a **decade** away.

Word list

(to) lend	prêter
plea	appel / plaidoyer
scientist	chercheur
proof of principle	validation de principe
grade	qualité / type
(to) behave	se comporter
(to) scale up	passer à l'échelle / à la vitesse supérieure
(to) sound	paraître
eligible	répondant aux critères
willing	consentant
concern	inquiétude / crainte
IVF (in-vitro fertilization)	FIV (fécondation in-vitro)
(to) raise	soulever
(to) overcome	surmonter
self-renewing	auto-régénérant
Holy Grail	quête ultime / Saint Graal
leap	avancée considérable / bond en avant
decade	décennie

ADDITIONAL VOCABULARY

blood test	prise de sang
(to) take a blood sample	faire une prise de sang
(to) draw blood	prélever du sang
on an empty stomach	à jeun
fasting glucose	glycémie à jeun
blood group	groupe sanguin
type O blood	sang de groupe O
blood typing	détermination du groupe sanguin
blood sugar / glycaemia	glycémie
diabetes blood test	test de dépistage du diabète
blood cholesterol test	test de dépistage du cholestérol
iron deficiency	carence en fer
anaemia	anémie
blood urea nitrogen (BUN)	urée sanguine
blood alcohol level (BAL)	taux d'alcoolémie

sexually-transmitted diseases blood test	test de dépistage MST
HIV test	test VIH
compatibility	compatibilité
blood bank	banque du sang
blood bag	poche de sang
blood unit	unité de sang
blood gases	gaz du sang
cord blood	sang de cordon

TRANSLATION

1. Written translation: Translate the following introduction of a research article into French.

Postpartum haemorrhage (PPH) is the principal cause of maternal death (21%) in France and is also responsible for considerable morbidity: anaemia, hypovolemic shock and disseminated intra-vascular coagulation.

It is defined as genital haemorrhage of more than 500 ml for vaginal delivery and more than 1000 ml for C-section.

Early diagnosis is necessary to implement preventive and curative measures, principally blood transfusion, as soon as possible to avoid the risks associated with delay. Estimations of blood loss are, however, often subjective, and it has been shown that such estimations are often too low.

The aim of this study was to evaluate the validity of an underbuttocks collection pouch in the diagnosis of PPH.

2. Translate the following passage into English.

L'anémie de Fanconi se caractérise par un dysfonctionnement de la moelle osseuse d'origine héréditaire.

Elle frappe les deux sexes et se manifeste chez les enfants de 5 à 10 ans par l'association de plusieurs signes cliniques : ralentissement de la production de globules rouges par la moelle et diverses malformations.

La maladie débute par une anémie progressive provoquée par une diminution des globules rouges, un manque de globules blancs et des hémorragies provoquées par un manque de plaquettes. Il en résulte des malformations telles que petite taille, anomalies des pouces, crâne peu développé, visage triangulaire, pigmentation brune de la peau, malformations rénales et génitales.

La greffe de moelle ou de sang de cordon, permet la survie du patient mais ne corrige pas les malformations ou le développement éventuel de cancers.

PAIR WORK

Using the pictures at the end of the book (**File 8**, p. 164), **student 1** explains to **student 2** how to apply a tourniquet and take a blood sample.

Chapter 22

TAKING CARE OF THE ELDERLY / SOINS AUX PERSONNES AGEES

NURSING SKILLS: ASSISTING WITH A BATH

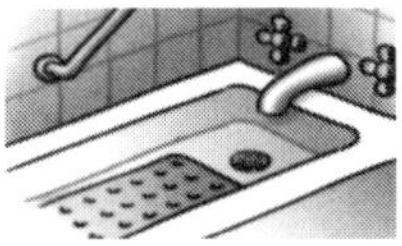

Place the bath **mat** in the **tub** and test the water.

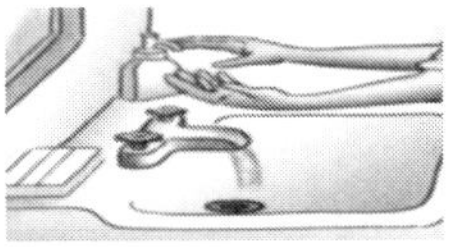

Wash and carefully dry your hands.

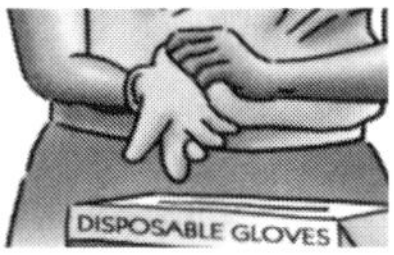

Put on your **disposable** gloves.

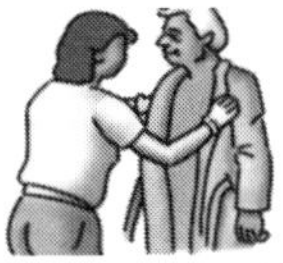

Help your patient undress.

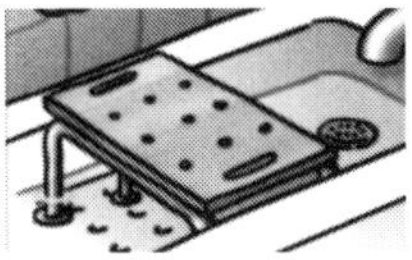

If your patient is not strong **enough** to stand, use a bath **stool**.

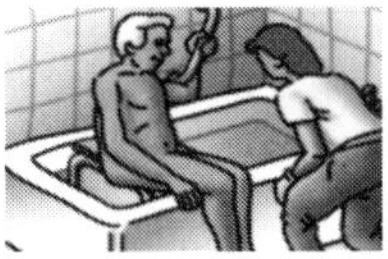

Help your patient sit on the edge of the tub.

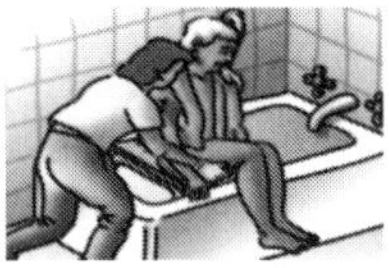

Swivel and lift both legs into the tub.

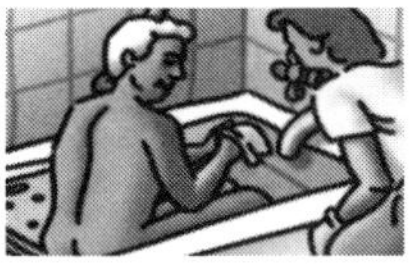

Encourage the patient to do as much for himself.

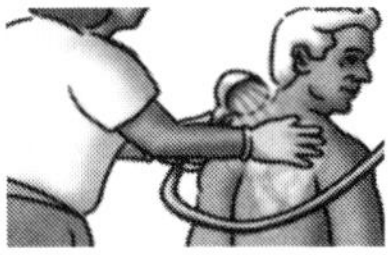

Assist the patient when necessary.

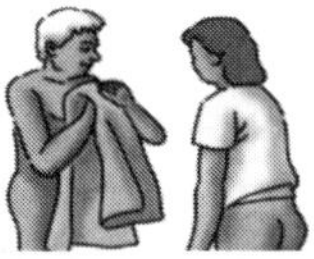

Help the patient dry his **upper** body.

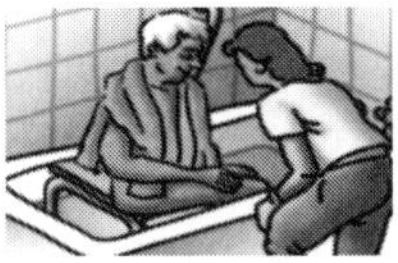

Let the water out of the tub and help the patient sit on the edge of the tub.

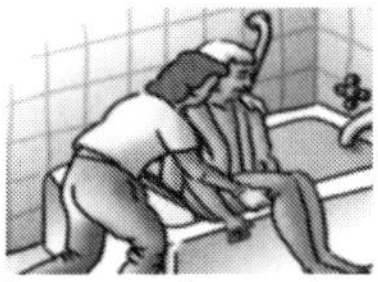

Support the patient and help him swivel his legs over the edge of the tub.

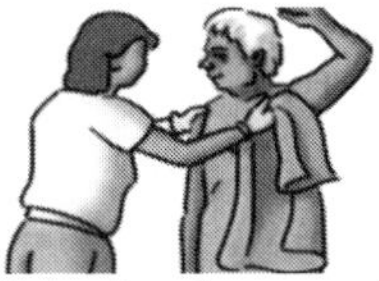

Help dry the rest of the body.

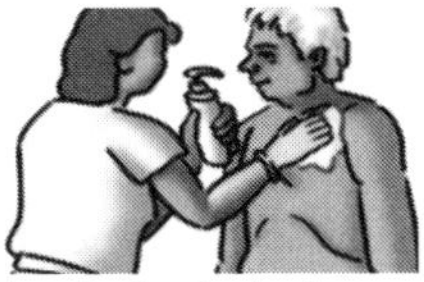

Apply body lotion to the skin and help the patient **dress**.

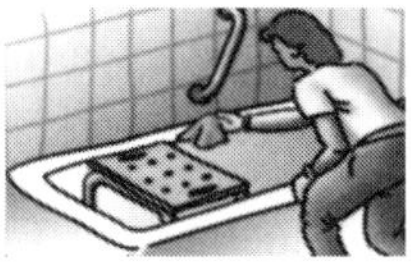

Return to the bathroom, clean the tub and **mop** the **floor**.

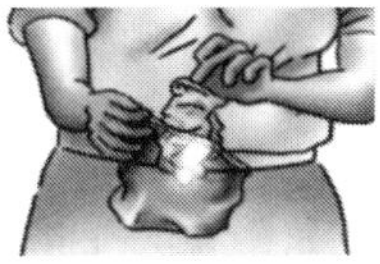

Remove the gloves and discard them in the disposable bag.

Word list

mat	tapis (de bain)
tub	baignoire
disposable	jetable
enough	assez / suffisamment
stool	tabouret (de bain)
(to) swivel	(faire) pivoter
upper	supérieur
(to) dress	s'habiller
(to) mop	passer la serpillère / essuyer
floor	sol

VIDEO

Choosing a **nursing home**

http://www.youtube.com/watch?v=6S8MXsDxsN0

Script:
Three months after entering a nursing home following a stroke, Janet once again walks with assistance.
Unidentified female: Left, right. Oh, I am doing good.
Unidentified female: You are doing **wonderful**.
Blakey: She remembers family and loves reading.
Unidentified female: This is gonna be a murder mystery.
Unidentified male: It is?
Unidentified female: Yes.
Unidentified male: You know I love you.
Unidentified female: I love you too.
Unidentified male: You're getting a kiss. I don't care.
Unidentified male: One of the places we went to, it looked like God's **waiting room**. They were really, really old, and they required so much help. Another place we went to there was 140 something patients there and they only had two therapists.
Blakey: We are at Keswick Multi Care Center in Baltimore Maryland, **once** known as the home for incurables. As a reporter who has been to a number of nursing homes, I must admit, Keswick does seem to **stand out** as a model of quality care.
(voice-over): **Still**, the quality of care can vary **widely** among the nation's nursing homes. In a first-of-its-kind program, the government's Centers for Medicare and Medicaid Services is publishing information measuring specific markers of care, **holding** nursing homes **accountable** for quality.
Tom Scully: We really believe that it's easier to find a restaurant than it is to find a good nursing home, and patients and their families, and you know, need more information about quality nursing homes. That's really the goal.
Blakey: A pilot program begins immediately in six states. Quality-of-care measures are **available** at www.medicare.gov for nursing homes in Maryland, Ohio, Rhode Island, Florida, Colorado and Washington State.

Libby Bowerman: I think that the **average** person who is looking for a nursing home for themselves or for their loved one will begin to have some information they can compare one nursing home to another.
Blakey: Improvement in walking is one of three measures used to **rate** short-term stays. Pain management and how often patients show signs of delirium are the other two. Measures for longer stays include things like infections, weight loss and bedsores.
As executive director of Keswick, Libby Bowerman likes the fact **raw numbers** will be adjusted to **level out the playing field**.
Bowerman: For example, at Keswick, we have met a lot of individuals who already have **skin breakdowns**. The risk adjustment will prevent us from looking like we have developed those within our **facility**.
Unidentified female: We are very supportive of this. We think that it is a very **bold** step for the administration and for long-term care, one that is long **overdue**.
Blakey: Still, there is no substitute for getting into the nursing home to visit where you can use your own senses of how the place looks, whether it is clean or not, how it smells, and the **friendliness** of the staff.

Word list

nursing home	maison de retraite médicalisée / EHPAD
wonderful	merveilleux / formidablement bien
waiting room	salle d'attente
once	autrefois
(to) stand out	se distinguer
still	néanmoins / toutefois
widely	largement
(to) hold accountable	tenir responsable de
available	disponible
average	moyen
(to) rate	évaluer
raw number	chiffre brut
(to) level out the playing field	mettre sur un pied d'égalité
skin breakdown	lésion cutanée
facility	établissement
bold	audacieux / courageux
overdue	attendu depuis longtemps
friendliness	gentillesse

ADDITIONAL VOCABULARY

quality of life (QOL)	qualité de vie
activities of daily living (ADL)	activités de la vie quotidienne
free-living	indépendant
aging	vieillissement
frail	frêle / fragile
weak	faible
walking frame / Zimmer frame	déambulateur

impairment	altération / dégradation
memory	mémoire
memories	souvenirs
memory loss	perte de mémoire
long-term memory	mémoire des faits anciens
short-term memory	mémoire des faits récents
food intake	prise alimentaire
undernutrition	sous-alimentation
dietary supplements	compléments alimentaires

TRANSLATION

Written translation: Translate the following extract from the introduction section of a research article into French.

As they get older, men and women eat less, have a poorer appetite and sometimes make inappropriate food choices. Due to this decline in food intake and loss of motivation to eat, people over 70 years of age often lose weight. In free-living elderly people, the prevalence of malnutrition induced by the decreased intake is relatively low (5-10%), but is considerably higher (30-50%) in hospitalized or institutionalized elderly people and could have serious adverse effect on health recovery.

Several studies have shown that taste and smell perception is seriously impaired, not only because of aging alone, but also because of disease and the consequent use of medications.

In order to increase food intake, high-energy, high protein supplements have often been used to enhance flavor and prevent weight loss and undernutrition in nursing homes, and several studies have shown that the use of supplements in hospitalized frail elderly people may increase energy and protein intake, even though less than 30% of the increased energy and protein intakes were provided by the supplements. To date, however, the impact of dietary supplements during periods of infection and convalescence remains unknown.

The aim of this study, therefore, was to determine whether or not such supplements could improve the health status of hospitalized frail elderly patients with infectious disease.

Consequently, we designed this study in hospitalized frail elderly patients with an infectious disease; firstly, to examine the impact of different taste modifications on taste pleasure and then on taking supplements, and secondly, to measure the impact of these flavor modifications on food intake. The study was conducted during both acute illness and convalescence in each patient.

PAIR WORK

Using the pictures at the end of the book (**File 9**, p. 164), **student 1** explains to **student 2** how to help an elderly patient to have a bath.

Chapter 23

ASSISTING THE SURGEON AND POST-OPERATIVE CARE / L'AIDE OPERATOIRE ET LES SOINS POST-OPERATOIRES

NURSING SKILLS: HELPING THE PATIENT GET OUT OF BED AFTER SURGERY

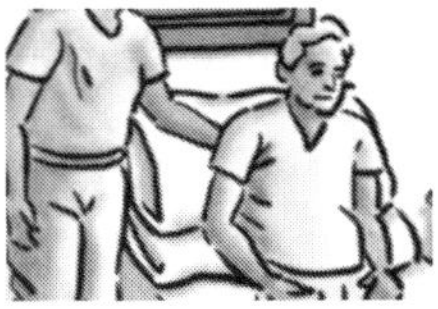

Always make the patient **sit up** for a few minutes.

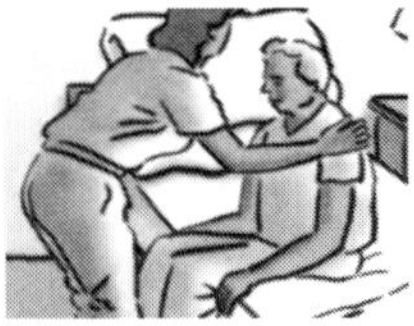

Sit the patient with legs **dangling** over the side of the bed.

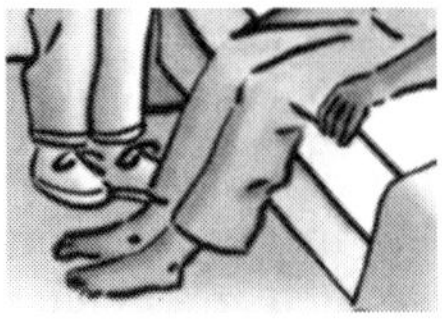

Instruct the patient to gently **swing** legs **back and forth.**

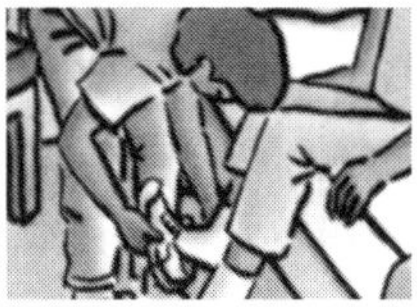

Help the patient put shoes or **slippers** on.

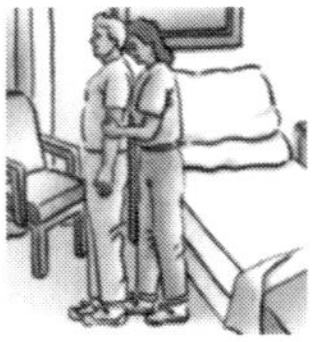

Make the patient **stand still** on the floor with feet slightly **apart**.

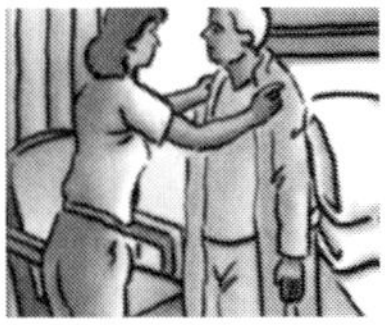

Put on and **fasten** the patient's **robe**.

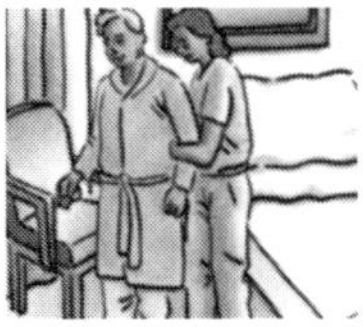

Make the patient walk a few **steps** towards a chair with **arms**.

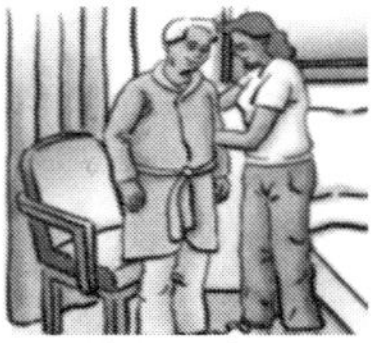

Turn the patient and help to **lower himself** backward into the chair.

Word list

(to) sit up	s'asseoir bien droit
(to) dangle	pendre
(to) swing	balancer / basculer
back and forth	d'avant en arrière
slippers	pantoufles
(to) stand still	se tenir immobile
apart	écarté
(to) fasten	attacher
robe	robe de chambre
step	pas
arm	accoudoir
(to) lower oneself (into the chair)	se laisser glisser / s'asseoir

VIDEO

The scrub nurse

http://www.youtube.com/watch?v=MpU6_rX9NQM&feature=related

Script:
Journalist: The scrub nurse assists the surgeon and maintains all materials within the **sterile field** that **surrounds** the patient during surgery.
Nurse: The scrub nurse first goes to the scrub **sink** where she'll **scrub** her arms from **2 inches** above the elbow down to the fingertips.
Journalist: Then, the nurse enters the **operating room**, and **dons** a sterile **gown**, gloves and **face mask** before preparing the sterile field. Anyone and anything allowed in this **germ-free** zone has been **thoroughly** sterilized.
Nurse: You have instruments, sponges and needles. All these things will be counted before, during, and at the **closure** of the surgery to make sure that nothing has been **retained** in the patient.
Journalist: The scrub nurse needs technical **knowledge** of the operation to anticipate what the doctor will need to keep the procedure moving forward.
Nurse: When I first **graduated** from **college**, I worked on a medical **surgical floor** and learned technical skills that I use here every day in the **OR**.

Word list

sterile field	champ stérile
(to) surround	entourer
sink	évier
(to) scrub	laver / désinfecter
2 inches	2 pouces (5 centimètres)
operating room (OR)	salle d'opération / bloc opératoire
(to) don	enfiler
gown	sarrau / blouse
face mask	masque chirurgical
germ-free	stérile / aseptisé
thoroughly	méticuleusement
closure	fermeture
(to) retain	oublier / laisser
knowledge	savoir / connaissances
(to) graduate	obtenir un diplôme / une licence
college	institut universitaire
surgical floor	département de chirurgie

ADDITIONAL VOCABULARY

surgeon	chirurgien
surgical procedure	intervention chirurgicale
reconstructive surgery	chirurgie réparatrice
keyhole surgery	chirurgie endoscopique / cœlioscopie
(to) operate on a patient	opérer un patient
operating theatre (GB)	salle d'opération / bloc opératoire
(to) perform an operation	effectuer une opération
(to) monitor	surveiller
anaesthesia (GB) / anesthesiology (US)	anesthésie
anaesthetist (GB) / anesthesiologist (US)	anesthésiste
operating table	table d'opération
suction	aspiration
ventilator	respirateur / ventilateur
hemostat	hémostat
instrument trolley (GB) / instrument cart (US)	chariot à instruments chirurgicaux
scrubbing	lavage chirurgical des mains
recovery room	salle de réveil
thread	fil
blade	lame
lancet / scalpel	lancette / scalpel
graft	greffe / greffon
flap	lambeau / volet / greffe

TRANSLATION

1. Translate the following sentences into English.

1. Les chirurgiens ont pu procéder à l'ablation de la vésicule biliaire par cœlioscopie.
2. Le lavage chirurgical des mains est une procédure obligatoire pour les chirurgiens et les infirmières de bloc avant d'entrer dans la salle d'opération.
3. L'instrumentiste a obtenu son diplôme à l'Institut Universitaire de Londres en 2007.
4. Si l'infirmier n'avait pas compté les compresses sur le chariot avant la fermeture de l'incision, le chirurgien en aurait laissé une dans l'abdomen du patient.
5. Pour que le champ stérile soit bien aseptisé, il faut que les instruments soient désinfectés méticuleusement.

2. Written translation: Translate the following extract from the introduction section of a research article into French.

In France, breast reconstruction using the latissimus dorsi flap, whether autologous or associated with an implant, is now the standard procedure following radical mammectomy for breast cancer.

The indications and the esthetic results are now well known. The principal aim of this so-called reconstructive surgery is not only to improve the woman's body image, but also indirectly her health-related quality of life in its physical, social, psychic and sexual dimensions. The efficacy of the management of cancer must be based on two main judgment criteria: survival and health-related quality of life. This multidimensional measurement is recognized as the main judgment criterion by the Food and Drug Administration (FDA) and the American Society of Clinical Oncology (ASCO).

However, there are no data in the literature that make it possible to judge the efficacy of this type of surgery in terms of improvement in quality of life.

We propose here to evaluate, on the one hand, the characteristics of patients who benefit from breast reconstruction and, on the other hand, the satisfaction of these women with reconstructed breasts by quantifying the impact of the reconstruction on their body image and quality of life.

PAIR WORK

Using the pictures at the end of the book (**File 10**, p. 165), **student 1** explains to **student 2** how to help a patient get out of bed after surgery.

Troisième année

S5-S6

Chapter 24

THE PAEDIATRIC NURSE / L'INFIRMIÈRE EN PÉDIATRIE

DOCUMENT FOR NURSES: THE RECORD CHART

WARD :	GP:
	REASON FOR ADMISSION:
SURNAME :	ADMISSION DATE:
CHRISTIAN NAME :	DIET:
DOB: AGE :	ALLERGIES:
GENDER:	SIZE: WEIGHT:

DATE (DDMMYY)										
TIME										
NURSE'S NAME										
T										
P										
RR										
BP										
ECG										
MEDICATION GIVEN										

Word list

T (temperature)	température
P (pulse)	pouls
RR (respiratory rate)	fréquence respiratoire
BP (blood pressure)	tension artérielle

VIDEO

Vital signs in children

http://www.youtube.com/watch?v=wio5qieaQaQ

Script:

What about children's vital signs? Just like for adults, the measurement of vital signs, an important **component** of assessment, includes a heart **rate**, respiratory rate, blood pressure and body temperature. But you have to remember that the normal parameters for children will vary according to size and age. Other factors that can affect measurement of vital signs in children include emotional state, overall physical condition, the equipment used, how it is used, movement and any **underlying disorders**. Heart rate is measured apically for infants and small children, and for all children you should count for a full minute. Tachycardia is a common sign indicating acute illness or stress. Bradycardia usually reflects poor airway control, so it requires immediate attention and possibly **CPR**. Respiratory rate should also be counted for a full 60 seconds. You must also observe respiratory effort and note any signs of respiratory distress. Blood pressure measurement can be affected by a variety of factors, time of day, age, gender, size activity level, medications, emotional state, physical condition and equipment used. Usually, blood pressure is measured in the upper arm or the lower leg. It's very important to use the correct size cuff? The **cuff bladder** should cover three quarters of the child's upper arm and completely encircle the arm or leg with **overlapping.** It is important to remember that hypertension is a late sign of inadequate circulation in children, so it requires immediate intervention. Temperature is measured to identify the presence of fever, of course, but hypothermia is also very important when **caring for newborns**. Cold stress in a newborn can cause metabolic acidosis, respiratory distress and hypoglycemia. A rapid rise in temperature can cause febrile **seizures** in some children. When a child has a fever you document and report that finding, and implement care to reduce the fever to provide for the child's comfort and well-being.

Word list

component	paramètre / composant
rate	fréquence / taux
underlying	sous-jacent
disorder	maladie / trouble
CPR (cardiopulmonary resuscitation)	RCP (réanimation cardio-pulmonaire)
cuff bladder	partie gonflable du brassard
overlapping	chevauchement
(to) care for	prendre soin de
newborn	nouveau né
seizure	crise (épileptique)

ADDITIONAL VOCABULARY

Pg = pregnant	enceinte
Pg = pregnancy	grossesse
FT = full term	né à terme
FTND = full-term normal delivery	accouchement à terme normal
IUGR = intra-uterine growth retardation	retard de croissance intra-utérin
FTT = failure to thrive	retard de croissance
Wt = weight	poids
BW = birth weight	poids de naissance
LBW = low birth weight	faible poids de naissance
Lb = pound	livre (0,45 kg)
Ht = height	taille

ft = foot	30,48 cm
in = inch	2,54 cm
STD / STI = sexually-transmitted disease / infection	maladie / infection sexuellement transmissible
SIDS = sudden infant death syndrome	mort subite (inopinée) du nourrisson
SB = still birth	mort-né
MMR = measles, mumps and rubella	ROR = rougeole, oreillons, rubéole
HC = head circumference	périmètre de la tête
VZV = varicella zoster virus	virus varicelle-zona
CNS = central nervous system	système nerveux central
CSF = cerebrospinal fluid	liquide céphalorachidien
LP = lumbar puncture	ponction lombaire

TRANSLATION

Written translation: Translate the following structured abstract into French.

Objective. To further characterize the clinical features and search for possible causative factors of atrophoderma of prematurity.

Design. Data from sixteen premature infants with a diagnosis of atrophoderma seen at a single institution during a seven-year period were retrospectively studied.

Results. All sixteen infants were extremely premature (25 to 33 weeks), had a very low birth weight, and half of them were born after twin pregnancies. Atrophoderma was initially diagnosed between six weeks and five months of age. Localized flat atrophic skin patches later became raised and herniated. They were located in subclavicular or paraumbilical areas. Five infants had had ecchymoses prior to atrophic patches. In most infants, the atrophic patches occurred at the site where the monitoring leads were placed. Digestive tract involvement and abdominal distension were noted in infants with abdominal atrophoderma. The incidence of atrophoderma decreased after implementing measures to avoid excessive pressure on monitoring leads. On follow-up, all atrophoderma lesions persisted without healing.

Conclusion. Atrophoderma of prematurity may be more common than previously reported. Most cases appear to originate from ecchymoses induced by pressure from monitoring leads, especially for thoracic lesions, whereas other unknown factors may be involved in abdominal lesions. Atrophoderma patches tend to persist and may later cause disfigurement. Thus, they should be prevented by avoiding placement of leads in visible areas.

PAIR WORK

Student 1 passes on the information below about a case of bronchiolitis to **student 2**, who is replacing him or her.

Gemma, 11 months old, admitted two days ago.

On admission:	cynanosis (blue lips) fever (39°C) sneezing, runny nose dry cough wheezing feeding difficulties drowsy signs of dehydration
Initial treatment:	inhaled bronchodilators liquid paracetamol to bring down temperature IV liquids for dehydration oxygen
Responding to treatment:	taken off oxygen so keep an eye on O_2 Sat check complexion can drink now so take down IV line give water regularly look for signs of dehydration make sure patient breathing easily – if wheezing or coughing or any deterioration call doctor immediately check temperature regularly

The mother is present and may need reassurance from time to time.

Chapter 25

ADMINISTERING DRUGS / L'ADMINISTRATION DES MEDICAMENTS

DOCUMENT FOR NURSES: DRUG DELIVERY SYSTEMS

1. What Day & Night Nurse Capsules® do.

Day & Night Nurse **Capsules**® are used for the 24 hour relief of the major symptoms of **colds**, chills and **influenza**.
The day-time capsules contain three active ingredients. Paracetamol is a painkiller and reduces your temperature when you have a **fever**. Pseudoephedrine hydrochloride **unblocks** your nose and sinuses helping you to breathe more easily. Pholcodine is a **cough suppressant** that helps relieve **dry** or **tickly** coughs.
The night-time capsules also contain three active ingredients. Paracetamol is a painkiller and reduces your temperature when you have a fever. Promethazine hydrochloride is an antihistamine which dries up a **runny nose** and aids **restful** sleep. Dextromethorphan hydrobromide is a cough suppressant that helps relieve dry or tickly coughs.

2. Check before you take Day & Night Nurse Capsules®.

Do not take Day & Night Nurse Capsules®:

- If you have ever had an allergic reaction to paracetamol, pseudoephedrine hydrochloride, promethazine hydrochloride, pholcodine, dextromethorphan hydrobromide or any of the other ingredients,
- If you have high blood pressure (particularly if due to a tumour near the kidney), epilepsy, hyper excitability, **overactive** thyroid, **enlarged** prostate, heart, kidney or liver problems, diabetes, glaucoma, asthma, **bronchitis** or other similar respiratory problems,
- If you are taking tricyclic antidepressants or if you have taken monoamine oxidase inhibitors prescribed for depression in the last two weeks,
- If you are having a pregnancy test carried out on your urine,
- If you are under 12 years.

Do not take with any other paracetamol-containing products.
Do not take with any other **flu**, cold or decongestant product.

3. How to take Day and Night Nurse Capsules®.

DAY-TIME: swallow two orange/yellow capsules with a drink, every four hours, up to three doses during the day.
NIGHT-TIME: swallow two green/white capsules with a drink, **at bedtime**.

If you take too many capsules:
Immediate medical **advice** should be **sought** in the event of an **overdose**, even if you feel well, because of the risk of **delayed** serious liver damage.
If your symptoms persist, see your doctor.

4. Possible side effects.

After taking Day & Night Nurse Capsules®, you may experience nausea (**feeling sick**), vomiting (being sick) **diarrhoea** or constipation, stomach pain, headache, **ringing in the ears**, irritability, **nightmares**, loss of appetite, difficulty in **passing urine**, rapid heart rate, **shaking** and skin rashes.

Word list

capsule	gélule
cold	rhume
influenza / (the) flu	grippe
fever	fièvre
(to) unblock	dégager / déboucher
cough suppressant	antitussif
dry (cough)	(toux) sèche
tickly (cough)	(toux) irritante / d'irritation
runny nose	nez qui coule
restful	réparateur / paisible
overactive	hyperactif
enlarged	hypertrophié
bronchitis	bronchite
at bedtime	au coucher
advice	conseil(s)
(to) seek (sought, sought)	chercher
overdose	surdosage
delayed	à retardement / différé
(to) feel sick	avoir la nausée
diarrhoea	diarrhée
ringing in the ears	bourdonnements d'oreilles
nightmare	cauchemar
(to) pass urine	uriner
shaking	tremblement

VIDEO

Errors in medication

http://www.youtube.com/watch?v=2T7H41_Guqo

Script:
Nurses who are interrupted while administering medications to hospital patients are more likely to make errors according to research published in the April 26th **issue** of the Archives of Internal Medicine. Medication errors can occur in hospitals, because of human errors

such as a nurse accidentally administering the **wrong** dose of a **drug**. System problems such as having two drugs with names that sound **alike** and both happening together. Researchers from the University of Sydney observed 98 nurses while they administered medication over 4,000 times to over 700 patients at two hospitals. Errors in procedure for the preparation and administration of drugs were noted as they were made. And the nurses' actions were also compared against the patients' medical charts to determine whether they administered the **right** drug in the correct **fashion**. Both errors and interruptions were common. Interruptions occurred 53% of the time. Nurses failed to follow proper procedure when preparing and administering drugs **nearly** three quarters of the time. They made **mistakes with respect to** the drug itself, including which drug was administered and when and how it was given one quarter of the time. Interruptions increased these error rates by about 12%, and the more interruptions occurred, the more errors were made. Four interruptions doubled the risk that a serious error, one that could cause substantial **harm** to the patient, would be made. Today's research suggests that changes should be made to how hospitals wards are **run** so that nurses are less frequently interrupted when performing crucial tasks such as administering drugs.

Word list

issue	numéro
wrong	mauvais
drug	médicament
alike	semblable / similaire
right	bon
fashion	manière
nearly	presque
mistake	erreur / faute
with respect to	par rapport à
harm	mal
(to) run	gérer / diriger

ADDITIONAL VOCABULARY

harmful	nocif
harmless	inoffensif
adverse effects	effets indésirables
side effect	effet secondaire
od (omni die) = every day	tous les jours
qd (quaque die) = every day	tous les jours
uid (unum in die) = once a day	une fois par jour
bid (bis in die) = twice a day	2 fois par jour
tid (ter in die) = three times a day	3 fois par jour
qid (quarter in die) = four times a day	quatre fois par jour
qqh (quater hora) = every four hours	toutes les quatre heures
ac (ante cibum) = before meals	avant le repas

pc (postcibum) = after meals	après les repas
po (per os) = by mouth	per os / par voie orale
pr (per rectum)	par voie rectale
tab = tablet	cp = comprimé
gtt (guttae) = drop	goutte
tsp = teaspoonful	cuillère à café
tbs = tablespoonful	cuillère à soupe
ung (unguent) = ointment	pommade
sup = suppository	suppositoire

TRANSLATION

Written translation: Translate the following article into French.

One in three patients victim of error

A study found that errors in the injection of medication are not an isolated phenomenon but are universal. One of the most important findings of the study was that errors in injectable medication in ICUs occur everywhere, which demonstrates the complexity of caring for critically ill patients.

Overall, 861 errors affecting 441 patients were reported - 250 were the victim of only one error and 191 suffered more than one. Most errors concerned antimicrobial drugs and sedation or analgesia.

Three quarters of the errors were classified as errors of omission. In most cases, these omissions had no significant impact on the patients' condition. However, in some cases, the outcome of patients exposed to such errors was very serious. According to the study, 12 patients experienced permanent harm or died because of errors of administration of medication. In particular, five died and seven were caused lasting harm, partly due to errors related to the injection of medications.

One could presume that errors in the administration of medication occur in extreme conditions, i.e. during on call time. On the contrary 69% of them occurred in routine situations. Almost two thirds of the errors were due, according to the medical professionals themselves, to failure to administer a medication on time. These omissions seem to have a less harmful impact on patients. However, there were errors where the wrong drug was administered - mainly due to a change in labeling or packaging – or the wrong dose of the drug. These errors can have a more serious impact on the health of patients. Medical staff stated that workload, stress and fatigue were the reasons behind the omissions, which in some cases may even cause death.

PAIR WORK

1. **Student 1** works with **student 2**. They match the following pictures with the following words, then insert them in the sentences below.

capsule / eye drops / inhaler / injection / nasal spray / ointments / suppository / syrups / tablets - pills

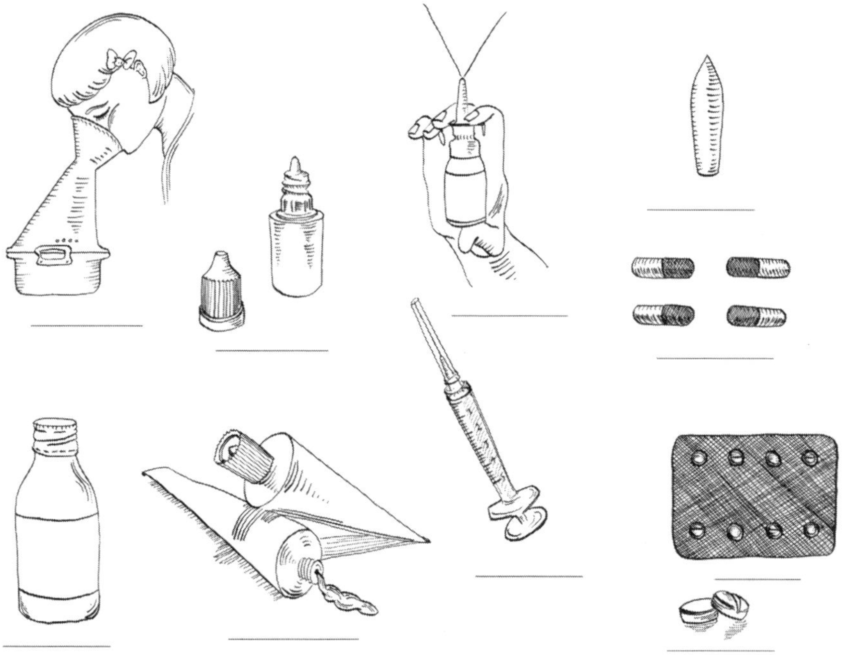

1. An _________ is a portable device often used to treat asthma. As it delivers the drug into the lungs, patients have to breathe in deeply when they use one.
2. A method of infusion that involves putting a drug into a vessel or a muscle via a needle and a syringe is called an _________.
3. In a _________, the active ingredient is contained in a soluble gelatinous case. It has to be swallowed without chewing.
4. By using _________ _________ it is possible to deliver drugs via the eye.
5. Because _________ are greasier than creams and have a thicker texture, they are able to adhere to the affected area longer.
6. _________ are liquids that have to be swallowed. They are generally sweet or flavoured and are used to treat coughs, for example.
7. _________ contain a precisely measured dose of a drug and are taken orally. They are usually sold in blister packs and are thus easy to carry around and use.
8. A _________ _________ is inserted into the nose to deliver drugs to relieve the symptoms of colds and allergies.
9. A _________ is a drug-delivery system administered through the rectum.

2. Using the abbreviations and the words above, **student 1** explains to **student 2** what medications he/she must take, which ointment he/she must use …when and how often.

Ex. Tab pc tid
Student1 to **student 2** (patient)
Don't forget to take these pills / tablets 3 times a day after meals.

- Apply ung bid
- Put sup pr every evening
- Take 1 tbs cough syrup qqh
- 4gtt each eye tid

…
Now, create your own…

Chapter 26

THE PSYCHIATRIC NURSE / L'INFIRMIERE EN PSYCHIATRIE

DOCUMENT FOR NURSES: ANTIDEPRESSANTS

Why have I been prescribed an **antidepressant**?
Antidepressants can be used to help treat depression, **generalised anxiety disorder**, **obsessive compulsive disorder**, **panic disorder**, **social phobia**, **post-traumatic stress disorder** and **bulimia nervosa**.
Are antidepressants safe to take?
Let your **prescriber** know if any of the following apply to you:

- Epilepsy, diabetes, heart, liver or kidney trouble,
- If you take any other medication including medication bought over the counter and alternative therapies,
- If you are pregnant or **breast-feeding** or **wish** to become pregnant.

Antidepressants can take up to 4-6 weeks (eight weeks in people older than 65) to produce their full benefits in depression and can take up to 12 weeks in other conditions, **e.g.** anxiety disorders. Antidepressants are then continued for a minimum of six months **once** your **condition** has improved. Antidepressants may be needed for longer but your doctor will discuss this with you.
Antidepressants should be continued even if you feel well as they reduce the risk of you becoming unwell again. Antidepressants work in different ways and so, if the first drug does not suit you, another may be effective.
All antidepressants may **cause** an increase in anxiety, agitation, suicidal ideas and **restlessness** initially. These side-effects should improve after the first 1-2 weeks. If they are still problematic, then please discuss them with a healthcare professional.

Word list

antidepressant	antidépresseur
generalised anxiety disorder	troubles de l'angoisse généralisés
obsessive compulsive disorder (OCD)	trouble obsessionnel compulsif (TOC)
panic attacks	crises d'angoisse
panic disorder	trouble panique
social phobia	phobie sociale
post-traumatic stress disorder (PTSD)	état de stress post-traumatique
bulimia nervosa	boulimie nerveuse
prescriber	médecin prescripteur
(to) breast-feed	allaiter

(to) wish	souhaiter / désirer
e.g.(= exempli gratia)	par exemple
once	une fois que
condition	état / maladie
(to) cause	provoquer
restlessness	agitation

VIDEO

Schizophrenia

http://www.youtube.com/watch?v=G6nhtpZjmW8

Script:
Schizophrenia affects about 1% of the US population. But what exactly is it? People with schizophrenia may hear voices or believe that other people are reading their **minds**, controlling their **thoughts** or **plotting** against them. These experiences are terrifying and can cause **fearfulness**, **withdrawal** or extreme agitation. Many schizophrenics do not make sense when they talk, sometimes **displaying** what is known as "word salad".
Eugen Bleuler first **coined** the term schizophrenia in 1911 and defined the disorder with his four As. **Blunted** affect or diminished emotional response, loosening of associations or reduced understanding of relationships, ambivalence, an **inability** to make decisions, and autism, a preoccupation with one's **own** thoughts and reduced awareness of external **events**. The psychotic symptoms associated with schizophrenia, hallucinations and **delusions**, tend to emerge earlier in men than in women. For men, symptoms appear in the late adolescence to mid twenties, while for women, schizophrenia's symptoms surface in the mid twenties to early thirties. The cause of schizophrenia is not known. But the **illness** is thought to **arise** from a combination of **inherited** and environmental factors. One percent of the general population is affected by schizophrenia. If one parent or **sibling** has schizophrenia, your chance of developing it is about 6%. If **both** parents have schizophrenia, your chance of developing it jumps to about 46%. When one identical **twin** is schizophrenic, the other has a 48% chance of developing it as well. People who have schizophrenia abuse alcohol and drugs more often than others. Substance abuse can make psychotic symptoms more severe. Although schizophrenia is a serious illness, the **outlook** for those diagnosed with the disorder has improved over the last thirty years. There's still no cure but effective treatments have been developed and many people with schizophrenia improve enough to **lead** independent satisfying lives. If someone you love has symptoms of schizophrenia, consult a mental health professional.

Word list

mind	esprit
thought	pensée
(to) plot	comploter
fearfulness	crainte
withdrawal	repli sur soi
(to) display	présenter
(to) coin	inventer / créer
blunted	émoussé

inability	incapacité
own	propre à soi / personnel
event	événement
delusion	délire
illness	maladie
(to) arise (from)	provenir (de)
inherited	génétique / hérité
sibling	frère ou sœur
both	les deux
twin	jumeau
outlook	perspectives
(to) lead	mener

ADDITIONAL VOCABULARY

a psychiatrist	un psychiatre
anorexia nervosa	anorexie mentale
mood disorder	trouble de l'humeur
mood swings	sautes d'humeur
melancholy	mélancolie
paranoia	paranoïa
paranoid	paranoïaque
attention deficit hyperactivity disorder (ADHD)	trouble d'hyperactivité avec déficit de l'attention (THADA)
psychosis	psychose
psychotic	psychotique
post-partum psychosis	psychose puerpérale
nervous breakdown	dépression nerveuse
self-esteem	estime de soi / amour propre
burnout	surmenage / épuisement
self-inflicted wound	automutilation

TRANSLATION

1. Written translation: Translate the following information sheet into French.

TYPES OF MENTAL ILLNESS

The following descriptions are brief. Further information can be obtained from voluntary and statutory mental health services, book shops, libraries and the Internet.

PSYCHOSIS:

This word is often misunderstood. It means the inability to distinguish between what is real and what is imagined. Three of us in every hundred people have this illness, which is more likely to affect young adults. With this disorder there is an impairment of our thoughts, emotional response and ability to communicate to others. We may hear voices or have beliefs (delusions) that make no sense to those who know us well. Alcohol and drug abuse can trigger psychotic episodes.

BIPOLAR AFFECTIVE DISORDER (Manic Depression):
This can include periods of low moods (depression) as mentioned and can alternate with ones of elation (being high). When we are high, we may have decreased need for sleep, increased speech, engage in inappropriate behavior or even become psychotic. About one of us in every two hundred has this illness. Medication usually has an important part in keeping us well and maintaining a level mood.

2. Written translation: Translate the following abstract into English.
La relation des soignants en psychiatrie : « La part de l'autre, la part de soi »

Résumé :
Aspirant à devenir cadre de santé en psychiatrie, il m'a semblé fondamental d'avoir une autre approche de la relation dans ce domaine du soin, tant dans le rapport soignant-soigné qu'au sein de l'équipe soignante. Au travers d'apports conceptuels et d'entretiens semi-directifs, j'ai cherché à mettre en lumière différents phénomènes permettant de caractériser ces échanges intersubjectifs. Le soin se définit alors dans une présence à l'autre par une présence à soi. Mais, considérant toute relation comme dialogique, cette présence peut s'avérer ardue dès lors que ce qui est vécu de la relation touche le soignant dans ses restrictions. Si le collectif de soins est alors une ressource, il peut être aussi le lieu de tension et de conflits, rendant mal aisé le soin au patient. Il revient au cadre de santé de porter son attention sur ce qui est vécu de la relation, tant dans l'interaction soignant-soigné que dans les interactions au sein de l'équipe soignante.

Mots clés : relation ; présence ; soin ; anthropologie de la folie.

PAIR WORK

Pair work: Split crossword puzzle
Student 1 looks at the crossword below, and **student 2** looks at the crossword in **File 11**, p. 165.
Student 1 asks **Student 2** for definitions or explanations of missing words.
Student 2 gives the definitions or the explanations without using the missing word.
Student 1 tries to find the word.
And vice versa, one word at a time.
This activity will give you the opportunity to practice the alphabet.

	a	b	c	d	e	f	g	h	i	j	k	l	m	n	o	p	q	r	s
1	B		E		S		-	F			D								
2	L		N		E			U			E								
3	I		T		I			N			L				B	L	O	O	D
4	S	N	E	E	Z	E		C		P	U	L	S	E					
5	T		R		U			T			S								
6	E		A		R			I			I	L	L	N	E	S	S		
7	R		L		E			O			O								
8			-	I				N			N		T			B	I	N	S
9			F	E		T					S								
10			E									A		T	W	I	N	S	
11			E		C							W							
12			D		O		S					A				G			
13			I		U		U					K							
14			N		G		G					E		D	R	A	I	N	
15	W	I	G		H	E	A	R	T	S							N	G	O
16					I		R										C		U
17		R			N												L		T
18		U			G												U		E
19		S							W	R	O	N	G				D		R
20	T	H	E	A	T	R	E										E		

Ex.

Student 1: What is a-15 across?

Student 2: It is something people who have lost their hair because of chemotherapy wear on their heads.

Student 1: Is it "wig"?

Student 2: That's right! What is b-7 down?

Student 1: It is the opposite of "on"

...

Chapter 27

PALLIATIVE CARE / LES SOINS PALLIATIFS

DOCUMENT FOR NURSES: BRIEF FATIGUE INVENTORY

We are interested in some things about you and your quality of life. Please answer all the questions yourself by **ticking** the **box** that best applies to you. There are no "right" or "wrong" answers. The information that you provide will remain strictly confidential.

	NOT AT ALL	A LITTLE	QUITE A BIT	VERY MUCH
Are you **in pain**?				
Do you have trouble sleeping?				
Do you feel weak?				
Have you lost your appetite?				
Do you feel nauseated?				
Does pain interfere with your **daily** tasks?				
Do you feel **tense**?				
Do you feel depressed?				
How **tired** do you feel?				
Do you feel **short of breath**?				
Are you satisfied with the **efficacy** of the treatment you are taking?				
Do you feel too much discomfort to enjoy the pleasant moments in your life?				
Do you accept the fact that you cannot do many of the things that you used to do?				

Word list

(to) tick	cocher
box	case
(to) be in pain	souffrir
daily	quotidien
tense	tendu
tired	fatigué
short of breath	essoufflé
efficacy	efficacité

VIDEO

Palliative care

http://www.youtube.com/watch?v=KF9lhL8dPJ4

Script:
Each year in the US, millions of people are hospitalized for a variety of reasons. Some are **admitted** through the ER, others admitted by their **physician** for surgery or some other form of medical treatment. But did you know that most people who **end up in** the hospital with **a serious** chronic illness will most likely require something called palliative care?
Diane Meier: Palliative care is medical care focused on the relief of pain and other symptoms, and support for the best possible quality of life for patients living with serious illness and for their families. And palliative care is delivered at the same time as all other medical care focused on prolonged life or curing disease.
The goal of palliative care is to relieve the pain, symptoms and stress of serious illness **whatever** the diagnosis or prognosis. It is appropriate for people of any age and at any point in an illness. It can be delivered along with treatments that are meant to cure you. Palliative care is typically provided by a **team** that includes palliative care doctors, nurses and social workers. The team works in partnership with your primary doctor.
Sue McHugh-Salera: Palliative care is a rapidly growing specialty. **Fortunately**, most larger hospitals in the United States offer a palliative care program. So patients who have a serious illness, who are having difficulty with symptoms, such as pain, nausea, vomiting can ask their doctor for a **referral**.
Palliative care is not a **one-size-fits-all approach**. A key benefit of palliative care is that it **customizes** treatment to **meet the needs** of each individual person.
Nathan Goldstein: I think that palliative care is right for a very **broad range of** patients. So it can be patients with diagnoses such as cancer, but certainly patients with any form of heart disease, lung disease, dementia, Parkinson's disease, any condition that has pain or any other symptom that **folks** will need help with **along the way**.
Diane Meier: Patients who are receiving palliative care report reduced pain and other distressing symptoms, and when they receive this care at the same time as their curative and life-prolonging treatments, they are better able to **handle** a **course of treatment** that their doctor has recommended for them.
Anna Loengard: My recent personal experience with palliative care was when I was in the hospital for a benign brain tumor and it really made me realize as a physician how important palliative care is, that despite the fact that I was being treated by world-class surgeons, that I really needed somebody who was specifically looking out for my other symptoms, my pain management, the nausea that I had post-operatively, people who weren't necessarily just interested in the incision that I had, and **whether** the surgery was a success, but really were looking at me as a whole individual, and people who could advocate for me in getting adequate pain management and other symptom management, that really is not the **forte** of surgeons even if they are world-class.

Word list

(to be) admitted to hospital	entrer / être admis à l'hôpital
physician (US)	médecin
(to) end up in	finir à
serious (illness)	(maladie) grave
whatever	quel que soit
team	équipe
fortunately	heureusement
referral	transfert / orientation (du patient)
one-size-fits-all approach	approche universelle
(to) customize	personnaliser
(to) meet the needs (of)	satisfaire les besoins (de)
broad range of	large éventail de
folks (US)	les gens
along the way	au cours de (la maladie...)
(to) handle	supporter
course of treatment	traitement
whether	si
forte	point fort

ADDITIONAL VOCABULARY

terminally-ill patient	patient en phase terminale
end of life	fin de vie
aggressive life-sustaining therapy / heroic treatment	acharnement thérapeutique
euthanasia	euthanasie
critically ill	gravement malade
life-threatening	qui engage le pronostique vital
accompaniment	accompagnement
counselling	soutien psychologique
physician-assisted suicide	suicide médicalement assisté
supportive care	soins de soutien
(to) cope with	faire face à

TRANSLATION

1. Put the words in the right order to form coherent questions, and then translate them into French.

1. regularly / activities / do you / to improve / engage in / your health?
2. see your GP / for changes / how / to check / often / in your health / do you ?
3. you know / your health problems / trigger / and make them worse / do / what can ?
4. your health problems / your life / are / unbearable / making ?
5. feel depressed / think about / do you / health problems / when / you / your?
6. or relatives / often / your home / to visit / you leave / do / how / friends?

2. Written translation. Translate the following QOL questionnaire into English.

INSTRUCTIONS:
Indiquez dans quelle mesure vous êtes d'accord ou non avec les propositions suivantes en cochant la réponse qui correspond le mieux à votre situation.
Il n'y a ni bonne ni mauvaise réponse. Si vous faites une erreur ou changez d'avis, merci de rayer la mauvaise réponse et de cocher la bonne.

SYMPTOMES

Je me sens mal en permanence.

Tout à fait d'accord	D'accord	Sans avis	Pas d'accord	Pas du tout d'accord

Je suis satisfait(e) de l'efficacité du traitement actuel de mes symptômes.

Tout à fait d'accord	D'accord	Sans avis	Pas d'accord	Pas du tout d'accord

Je suis trop gêné(e) physiquement pour profiter de moments agréables.

Tout à fait d'accord	D'accord	Sans avis	Pas d'accord	Pas du tout d'accord

ACTIVITÉS QUOTIDIENNES

Je ne suis plus capable de faire bon nombre de choses que j'aimais faire.

Tout à fait d'accord	D'accord	Sans avis	Pas d'accord	Pas du tout d'accord

J'accepte de ne plus pouvoir faire bon nombre de choses que je faisais auparavant.

Tout à fait d'accord	D'accord	Sans avis	Pas d'accord	Pas du tout d'accord

Mon bien-être est limité par ma capacité à être actif / active et indépendant(e) pour mes besoins personnels *(faire ma toilette, aller aux toilettes, m'habiller, manger…)*.

Tout à fait d'accord	D'accord	Sans avis	Pas d'accord	Pas du tout d'accord

PAIR WORK

Create a questionnaire about job satisfaction as a nurse and ask your partner your questions.

Ex.
Student 1: Where do you work?
Student 2: At the teaching hospital.
Student 1: Which department do you work in?
Student 2: At the OPD.
Student 1: What are your working hours?
…

Chapter 28

THE ICU NURSE / L'INFIRMIERE EN SOINS INTENSIFS

DOCUMENT FOR NURSES: THE ICU INFORMATION LEAFLET

In this **leaflet** we hope to help you understand our work by giving you some information about the Intensive Care/High Dependency **Unit**, the equipment we use and the people who work here.

Visiting

When visiting, we ask you to ring the **doorbell** to the right of the entrance doors and wait until a member of staff speaks to you through the intercom, which may take **a little while**, so please be patient.

Visiting times are: 2.00 pm till 8.00 pm **unless** there are **prior** arrangements with the person in charge. We also ask relatives to return home at night unless there are exceptional circumstances. We do have a sofa bed for those relatives who may occasionally need to stay overnight. Visiting is limited to **close** family only and two people at the bedside at any time to prevent tiring the patient. You may find that you are asked to wait outside for five minutes while procedures take place. This may well **stretch** to 15 minutes or longer so please be prepared to wait as we do try to get to see you as soon as we can!

There will be a qualified nurse with your relative 24 hours a day, who is available to answer questions at any time. We will always let you know how treatment is progressing and can arrange for the doctors to speak with the immediate family.

Storage space for clothing and **valuables** is limited so we ask the family to take home all **items of clothing** and valuables belonging to the patient; the only things patients will require are their usual toiletries.

Flowers

We ask visitors not to bring flowers as the water they are in often contains bacteria which can be harmful to very ill patients.

Given the nature of Intensive Care your relative will be **closely** observed by the use of a variety of monitors, lines and tubes. The nurse caring for your relative will be happy to explain about these, so please feel free to ask.

Daily Activities

An illustration of the everyday activities on the Intensive Care Unit might be:

07.00 hours: Morning **handover** – nurses **shift** changes

08.30 hours: Investigations

Morning bed baths

Doctor's **round**

Physiotherapy

X-rays

14.00 hours: Physiotherapy
Wound dressing
19.00 hours: Night handover – nurses shift change
20.00 hours: Evening bed bath

Word list

leaflet	brochure / dépliant
unit	unité / service
doorbell	sonnette
(a little) while	(un petit) moment
unless	à moins que
prior	précédent / antérieur
close	proche
(to) stretch	se prolonger
valuables	objets de valeur
item (of clothing)	article (vestimentaire)
given	étant donné
closely	étroitement / de près
handover	transmission
shift	équipe
(doctor's) round	visite (au chevet du malade)

VIDEO

ICU in Australia

http://www.youtube.com/watch?v=JX6D_3wY3xs

Script:
(voice off): You're in the intensive care unit and you've just had an operation…
We look after the **sickest** people in the hospital, and the most potentially sick patients…
Basically, they need a **range** of advanced nursing skills…
He is quite **unwell** at the moment, but it's nothing we can't deal with…
It's very high-cost, high-tech, high-acuity healthcare.
Journalist: Intensive care units look after the most seriously ill and dependent patients in the hospital. Patients are usually kept alive by a ventilator, a complex machine which breathes for the patient. Patients are unconscious and require **one-to-one nursing**. Without warning, a patient's condition can change from stable to life-threatening. Intensive care is a highly specialized area and it is an **area** in which Australia is the world leader.
In an effort to make sure our intensive care units remain world class, a foundation has been set up to support research in intensive care.
Dr Nerina Harley: The foundation was established in 1990. It's the Charity for Intensive Care, and directed **solely** at clinical research and **funding** clinical research, which directly goes towards patient care and improving **outcomes** and ultimately saving lives.

Word list

sick	malade
basically	au fond / en fait
range	éventail / gamme
unwell	souffrant / qui ne se sent pas bien
one-to-one nursing	soins individuels
area	domaine
solely	uniquement
(to) fund	financer
outcome	devenir / issue

ADDITIONAL VOCABULARY

trach. = tracheostomy / tracheotomy	trachéotomie
MV = mechanical ventilation	ventilation mécanique
ET = endotracheal tube	sonde d'intubation
EF = enteral feeding	alimentation entérale
RDS = respiratory distress syndrome	syndrome de détresse respiratoire
COPD = chronic obstructive pulmonary disease	BPCO = bronchopneumopathie chronique obstructive
ABG = arterial blood gases	gaz du sang artériel
PPV = positive pressure ventilation	ventilation à pression positive
NPV = negative pressure ventilation	ventilation à pression négative
V_t*= tidal volume*	volume courant
PIP = peak inspiratory pressure	PIP = pression inspiratoire de pointe
SaO_2 *= arterial oxygen saturation*	saturation du sang artériel en oxygène
PaO_2 *= partial pressure of oxygen in arterial blood*	pression en oxygène dans le sang artériel
PEEP = positive end expiratory pressure	pression positive en fin d'expiration
ARDS = acute respiratory distress syndrome	SDRA = syndrome de détresse respiratoire de l'adulte
BCLS = basic cardiac life support	maintien artificiel des fonctions cardiaques
ACLS = advanced cardiac life support	maintien artificiel amélioré des fonctions cardiaques
MOF = multiple organ failure	déficience polyviscérale
RF = renal failure	insuffisance rénale
CPR = cardiopulmonary resuscitation	réanimation cardio-pulmonaire

TRANSLATION

1. Written translation: Translate the following information leaflet into French.

Nursing care, such as frequent changes of position, eye and mouth care for your relative, is carried out throughout the 24-hour period.

We try to keep the next of kin informed of all aspects of a patient's condition and can arrange for them to be seen by a doctor if necessary. For reasons of confidentiality, we do not give detailed information over the telephone. Please arrange for one person to telephone on behalf of relatives or friends, so that they can then pass on this information to the others. Unfortunately, most of our patients are not well enough to make telephone calls but we can pass messages on if necessary.

It is important that all intensive care patients receive the highest quality care. To help do this, this intensive care unit is regularly assessed by an independent, charitable organisation. Information (or data) on every patient admitted to the unit is collected by unit staff and sent to this organisation. The organisation confidentially analyses the data and sends the results back to the unit. The health care team in this unit can use these results to improve the care they give their patients.

For further information, please ask for a leaflet.

2. Written translation: Translate the following abstract into English.

La mobilisation précoce des patients à l'hôpital et dans le service de soins intensifs est une pratique ancienne. Cependant, à une époque plus récente, une sédation profonde et un alitement ont fait partie des soins médicaux routiniers pour de nombreux patients ventilés mécaniquement. Un corpus grandissant de la littérature démontre que les survivants de réanimation présentent communément des complications neuromusculaires significatives et prolongées qui atteignent leur fonction physique et leur qualité de vie après la sortie de l'hôpital. L'alitement et ses mécanismes associés, peuvent jouer un rôle important dans la faiblesse neuromusculaire chez les patients en réanimation. Une nouvelle approche de la prise en charge des patients ventilés mécaniquement comprend la réduction de la sédation profonde et l'augmentation de la kinésithérapie et de la mobilisation tôt après l'admission en unité de soins intensifs. Les recherches récentes dans ce domaine apportent des preuves préliminaires corroborant la sécurité et les bénéfices potentiels de la mobilisation précoce en réanimation.

PAIR WORK

Using the ICU leaflet above, act out a dialogue between a visiting relative and the ICU nurse.

Ex.

Student 1: My husband / wife is a patient in the ICU, when can I visit him / her?

Student 2: Visiting times are from 2.00 pm till 8.00, but in exceptional circumstances, you can visit outside these hours if you ask the person in charge.

...

Chapter 29

THE ONCOLOGY NURSE / L'INFIRMIERE EN ONCOLOGIE

DOCUMENT FOR NURSES: CHEMOTHERAPY

Information leaflet

The word 'chemotherapy' means treatment with drugs. The word is used mostly to mean the treatment of cancer.

Sometimes the drugs used to treat cancer are called cytotoxic drugs. The word cytotoxic means poisonous or toxic to the cells of the body. Your chemotherapy treatment will depend on the type of cancer that you have. Different drugs work best on different cancers. Sometimes only one drug is required. Often more than one drug is used to make the treatment more effective. A **single** treatment may be given, or it may be repeated with a **rest** between each treatment. Sometimes, chemotherapy is used with surgery and / or radiotherapy to treat certain types of cancer.

How does chemotherapy work?

The drug will be given as tablets or capsules, or injected into a vein, so that it can enter your bloodstream. Tablets or capsules dissolve in your **gut** and the drug **passes through** the gut wall into your bloodstream. The drug is carried around your body in the bloodstream to reach the cancer cells. The drug gets into the cancer cells and may **damage** their genetic material (DNA). This may prevent the cancer cells from growing and dividing in an uncontrolled way. Cytotoxic drugs damage healthy cells as well, but the healthy cells are much more able to **recover** than the cancer cells. When healthy cells are affected, you may get temporary side effects, such as feeling sick, losing your hair, in which case you may need a wig, or getting a **sore** mouth. Usually, you will have your chemotherapy followed by a rest period, **e.g.** chemotherapy on one day and then 20 days rest period (this is then **referred to** as a cycle of chemotherapy). The rest period is most often longer than the chemo period. This rest or break is important as it gives your body's healthy cells time to recover from the **unwanted** effects of the treatment.

Word list

single	unique / seul
rest	repos
gut	intestin
(to) pass through	traverser
(to) damage	endommager
(to) recover	se régénérer / se rétablir / récupérer
(to) refer to	faire référence à
unwanted	indésirable

VIDEO

Introduction to the Oncology Nursing Society

http://www.youtube.com/watch?v=mC5-UDFzOr0

Script:
Journalist: According to recent statistics, more than 1.4 million new cases of cancer are diagnosed and treated in America each year. The majority of this care is provided in an **outpatient** setting or during relatively short **hospital stay**s administered and coordinated by **skilled**, caring oncology nurses.
Brenda Nevidjon: What patients and families may not know at first is that most of their care is gonna be provided in the outpatient setting **whether** they're receiving chemotherapy **or** radiation therapy, and they will be seeing nurses very **consistently throughout** their treatment phase.
Journalist: Brenda is president of the Oncology Nursing Society, an organization made up of over 37,000 registered nurses and other health care providers dedicated to promoting excellence in patient care, education and research in oncology nursing.
Paula Rieger: The vision of ONS is to lead the transformation of cancer care. By that we mean working collaboratively with other health care professionals to prepare the profession for the future. Oncology nurses serve to help patients and families navigate their way through a treatment and living with cancer. They make a difference in both administering treatments to patients, helping them to manage side effects, but a **critical** role that nurses play is helping to educate them about their disease, about their treatment and to cope with and manage life with cancer.
Linda Person: As a professional, you need to support the profession and yourself, and the Oncology Nursing Society allows you to grow as a nurse and to meet people from all around the world with similar issues and challenges. It's an ideal organization I truly do believe in.
Journalist: Learn more about the Oncology Nursing Society today where oncology nurses connect. Call (866) 257-4ONS, or visit ons.org for more information.

Word list

outpatient	(en) ambulatoire
hospital stay	séjour hospitalier
skilled	compétent / qualifié
whether ... or	que … ou que
consistently	régulièrement
throughout	tout au long de
critical	crucial / clé

ADDITIONAL VOCABULARY

biopsy	biopsie
benign	bénin
malignant	malin
adjuvant therapy	thérapie adjuvante
relapse	récidive
remission	rémission
port / portacath	cathéter à chambre implantable
organs at risk (OAR)	organes à risque
lumpectomy	chirurgie mammaire conservatrice
reconstruction surgery	chirurgie réparatrice
precancerous polyps	polypes précancéreux
(to) metastasize	métastaser
metastasis (pl. metastases)	métastase
lymph node	ganglion lymphatique
PET scan	TEP / PET
CAT scan	scanner
(to) respond to treatment	répondre au traitement
survival rate	taux de survie
disease-free survival	survie sans maladie
relapse-free survival	survie sans récidive
stage	stade
prognosis	pronostic

TRANSLATION

1. Written translation: Translate the following information leaflet into French.

Oncology Nurse Information

An oncology nurse cares for patients who are undergoing or recovering from cancer treatments. While this is a rewarding career, it can also be a difficult one. Oncology nurses deal with painful situations daily.

Client Ages

Patients that are cared for by oncology nurses can be of any age, from infants to the elderly.

Client Diagnoses

The patient may be in any stage of cancer, from diagnosis to terminal. They may be receiving chemotherapy or being treated for cancer side effects such as chronic pain.

Rewards

Some of the rewards of being an oncology nurse are being a strong support for the patient and patient's family and making a difference in their lives.

Difficulties

Difficulties include coping with death and pain, difficult patients, stressful environment and excessive paperwork.

Education

An oncology nurse is an RN with a Bachelor's degree. A Bachelor of Science in Nursing (BSN) is usually preferred.

Certifications and Associations

Oncology nurses can become certified through the Oncology Nursing Certification Corporation. They can also belong to the Association of Pediatric Oncology Nurses.

2. Written translation: Translate the following abstract into English.

L'annonce du diagnostic du cancer d'un enfant: sur le chemin de l'hospitalisation

L'annonce d'un cancer à un enfant et à ses parents est toujours un moment douloureux du fait du pronostic souvent défavorable associé à cette maladie et aux effets indésirables des traitements.

La prise en charge de l'enfant en hématologie-oncologie doit être globale et adaptée au plus près à ses besoins fondamentaux. L'annonce du diagnostic est le point de départ de cette prise en charge ; la faire dans de bonnes conditions permet de créer un climat de confiance avec cette famille.

Comment l'infirmier fait-t-il face à cette situation délicate ? Quel doit être son comportement tout au long du séjour hospitalier ?

Cette étude aborde l'importance de conserver une trace écrite de l'annonce du diagnostic, afin d'adapter la prise en charge globale de l'enfant.

Le rôle du médecin référent sera clarifié dans le but de mettre en place un projet de soins individualisés dans le cadre d'un travail d'équipe.

PAIR WORK

Explain to the parents of a child with cancer the regimen and side effects of the chemotherapy he or she will need.

Ex.

Student 1: Is chemotherapy the same treatment for everybody?

Student 2: No, it depends on the type of cancer a person has.

Student 1: How often will he need treatment?

…

Chapter 30

THE COMMUNITY NURSE / L'INFIRMIERE A DOMICILE

DOCUMENT FOR NURSES: DISTRICT NURSING

Role of a district nurse
District nurses play a crucial role in the primary health care team. They visit people in their own **homes** or in **residential care homes**, providing **ongoing** care for patients and supporting family members.
As well as providing direct patient care, district nurses also have a teaching role, working with patients to **enable** them to care for themselves or with family members teaching them how to give care to their relatives.
District nurses play a vital role in keeping hospital admissions and readmissions to a minimum and ensuring that patients can return to their own homes as soon as possible.
As a district nurse, you will assess the health care needs of patients and families, monitor the quality of care they're receiving and be professionally **accountable** for **delivery of care**. Your patients can be of any age, but often many of them will be elderly, while others may have been recently discharged from hospital, be terminally ill or have physical **disabilities**.
You may be visiting patients every day or more than once a day, offering help, advice and support. You may work on your own or with other groups, such as the social services, voluntary agencies and other **NHS** organisations and help to provide and co-ordinate a wide range of care services.
Skills required
You must be a qualified and registered nurse and will need to **undertake further training.** You will need to be **adaptable** and **resourceful**, working in a variety of workplaces and without the resources of a hospital **at hand.** You'll need to be well organised, **confident** and able to cope in potentially **challenging situations**.
Training
District nurse training programmes are known as specialist practitioner programmes and are at degree level. They are normally no less than one **academic year** (32 weeks) full time or part-time equivalent. They may be completed in a shorter period of time where credit is given for prior learning or experience.
Specialist practitioner programmes **comprise** 50% theory and 50% practice and concentrate on four areas:

- clinical nursing practice,
- care and programme management,
- clinical practice development,
- clinical practice **leadership.**

Community staff nurses can obtain **funding** for a district nurse specialist practitioner programme **via** their employing **trust hospital**. Alternatively, **applicants** with the **relevant** qualification and experience can **apply for** sponsorship via primary care trusts.

Word list

home	maison / foyer
residential care home	foyer / logement pour personnes âgées
ongoing	continu / suivi
(to) enable	permettre
accountable	responsable
delivery of care	administration des soins
disabilities	handicap
NHS (National Health Service) (GB)	branche maladie du régime de sécurité sociale britannique
(to) undertake	entreprendre
further	complémentaire/supplémentaire
training	formation
adaptable	souple / qui sait s'adapter
resourceful	plein de ressources / ingénieux
at hand	à proximité / à disposition
confident	confiant
challenging situation	situation difficile à surmonter
academic year	année universitaire
(to) comprise	comprendre
leadership	qualités de chef
funding	financement
via	par l'intermédiaire de
trust hospital (GB)	hôpital
applicant	candidat
relevant	pertinent
(to) apply for	faire une demande

VIDEO

Visiting Nurses

http://www.youtube.com/watch?v=wZAk0U6zTZk

Script:
Female journalist: Well, in Twelve on Health, you might say they're as **reliable** as letter carriers.
Male journalist: Visiting nurses say **trudging** through the elements is part of their job.
Female journalist: Right, well, here now is Twelve on Health reporter Gillian Neff, Gillian.

Gillian Neff: You **guys**, they are **troopers**. Lots of things get **cancelled** and **rescheduled** when the **weather** is **icy** like today, but when someone needs physical and mental health help, the nurses I spoke with today say they don't cancel.
Sharon Bradley: It's **tough** with the **snow** and the **ice** and the **sleet**.
Telephonist: Visiting Nurse and Hospice, Fairfield County – just **hold on** one second.
Gillian Neff: Some jobs can't be **put on hold** …due to dangerous winter weather.
Sharon Bradley: It is a balance between getting to the patients who need us **desperately**, sometimes **against the odds** of the weather.
Gillian Hansen: I'm **heading into** Newark to see a sixty-four-year-old female who has lung cancer and who is on oxygen.
Gillian Neff: Registered nurse Gillian Hansen has two little **kids** at home and **homebound** patients in southwestern Connecticut who count on her.
Sharon Bradley: Travelling and dealing with weather and dealing with **uncertainties**, that, that's part of it, but our **commitment** to our patients, it **overrides** all of those challenges.
Gillian Neff: Sharon Bradley, President of Visiting Nurse and Hospice of Fairfield County says nurses know…
Sharon Bradley: You have to be there for patients, **around the clock**. Visiting Nurses is all about that. Every day, we see 300 patients, and that might be someone who needs a nurse, that might be someone who needs a nurse's aide…
Gillian Neff: She says much of the visit is about medical care, but there's another health benefit that cannot be measured.
Sharon Bradley: The **companionship** of knowing that someone's coming out and **checking on** you and that is concerned about you **no matter what** the adversities might be or what the weather might be outside.
Gillian Neff: On Thursday, we will bring you Twelve on Health **coverage** of a high-tech method for helping patients who are homebound in southwestern Connecticut. Meanwhile, you can learn more about Visiting Nurses and Hospice of Fairfield County by going to our website, newstwelve.com.

Word list

reliable	fiable
(to) trudge	marcher péniblement / patauger
(you) guys	vous tous
troopers	(de vrais) soldats
(to) cancel	annuler
(to) reschedule	reprogrammer
weather	temps
icy	glacial
tough	dur / difficile
snow	neige
ice	glace / verglas
sleet	grésil
(to) hold on	patienter
(to) put on hold	mettre en attente
desperately	terriblement / désespérément
against the odds	contre les aléas
(to) head (into)	se diriger (vers)
kid	enfant / gamin
homebound	bloqué à la maison
uncertainties	aléas

commitment	engagement
(to) override	l'emporter sur
around the clock	24 heures sur 24
companionship	réconfort
(to) check on (somebody)	vérifier que quelqu'un va bien
no matter what	quel que soit
coverage	couverture (médiatique)

ADDITIONAL VOCABULARY

individually-tailored care	soins individualisés
wound care	soins des plaies
wound assessment	évaluation des plaies
leg ulcer care	soins d'ulcères de jambe
continence care	soins de la continence
end-of-life care	soins de fin de vie
drug delivery	administration des médicaments
route of administration / delivery route	voie d'administration
housebound	bloqué / confiné à la maison
long-term illness / long-term disease (LTD)	affection de longue durée
primary care	soins de première intention / de santé primaire
health education	hygiène publique
health visitor	infirmière des services sociaux
carer (GB)	accompagnant / aidant

TRANSLATION

1. Written translation: Translate the following information leaflet into French.

What is the District Nursing Service?

The District Nursing Service is a team which includes a Sister or Head Nurse, Staff Nurses and Health Care Assistants. They work closely with your General Practitioner and other Social and Health Care Professionals.

The District Nursing Service in Sunderland provides skilled nursing care and advice in a variety of health care settings. This includes treatment rooms, GP premises, residential homes and patients own home for those who are housebound.

How can we help you?

By providing:

• ongoing nursing care after leaving hospital,
• care for patients with long-term illness,
• expert specialist care when you are seriously ill,
• advice on how to live a more healthy life,
• health education and nursing care to aid recovery from illness,

• advice about continence services,
• referral to other specialist services as necessary,
• assessment for equipment to promote and maintain independence (e.g. wheelchair).

What you can expect from us?

The District Nursing Service will assess your individual health needs to provide skilled nursing care. You can expect the following from our service:

- to be treated as an individual,
- care delivered with respect, privacy and dignity,
- care provided by a named nursing team,
- individually-tailored care in which you and your carer have been involved in the planning and delivery of care,
- to have your care delivered by staff with the right skills to look after you.

2. Written translation: Translate the following abstract into English.

L'infirmière libérale (IDE) est au cœur de la prise en charge des soins des plaies des pieds diabétiques. La guérison dépendra de leurs connaissances et de leurs pratiques professionnelles.

Nous avons adressé un questionnaire à 50 IDE de notre département pour évaluer leur pratique concernant les soins de pied diabétique.

Dans leur clientèle, 44% des IDE ont entre 5 et 10 diabétiques (DT). Seulement 22% proposeront spontanément d'examiner les pieds de leurs patients. Deux-tiers des IDE ont un DT présentant une plaie de pied au moment du questionnaire. Seules 28% ont une ordonnance détaillée du protocole de soins (20% jamais) et le choix du pansement initial est effectué autant par l'IDE que le médecin généraliste (MG). L'évaluation de la plaie est visuelle chez 54% des IDE et 84% des IDE estiment avoir le matériel nécessaire à la réfection des pansements à domicile.

Ce questionnaire met en évidence les difficultés suivantes : absence de langage commun sur l'évaluation des différents types de plaie, absence de cohérence sur le soin spécifique, absence de coordination décisionnelle MG - IDE ou incompétence comme le déclarent 44% des IDE interrogées. La plupart réclament : les conseils d'un spécialiste (37%), une formation spécifique (30%), des consignes sur les pansements (22%), une ordonnance type (11%).

L'IDE libérale est un partenaire indispensable dans la prise en charge des plaies de pied diabétique. Ce soignant doit bénéficier d'une relation étroite avec les médecins généralistes et les diabétologues. Il faut définir des programmes de formation et organiser des transferts de compétences vers les soignants paramédicaux pour améliorer la prise en charge des plaies de pied des patients diabétiques.

PAIR WORK

Job interview

Student 1 has applied for a position as a community nurse for an English hospital.
Student 2 interviews the applicant.

Files / Annexes

File 1

STUDENT 2
Seven months
Followed husband
Loves children
Contact with families
Seriously ill children
Annual salary
Workload
Working hours
…

File 2

	a	b	c	d	e	f	g	h	i	j	k	l	m	n	o	p	q	r
1			-			-	C	-									-	
2	F	E	E	L	S		L						N				-	
3	-		-		M	-	O	-	-	-	D	-	U	-			-	
4	A	O	R	T	A		G		-		R		M		-		-	
5	-		-		L		G		-		U		B	R	E	A	S	T
6				B	L	-	E	-	-	-	G		N		-			
7				L			D		-		S	-	E	-	-			
8		-		O		M			-	I			S		-		A	
9	-	-	-	O	-	I	-			N			S	T	I	N	G	
10		-		D		L		-	-	S	-				-		R	
11		-				D				E			-	-	-	-	E	
12		-	-	-	-	E	-		D	R	I	P			-		E	
13						R				T								

File 3
SETTING UP AN I.V.

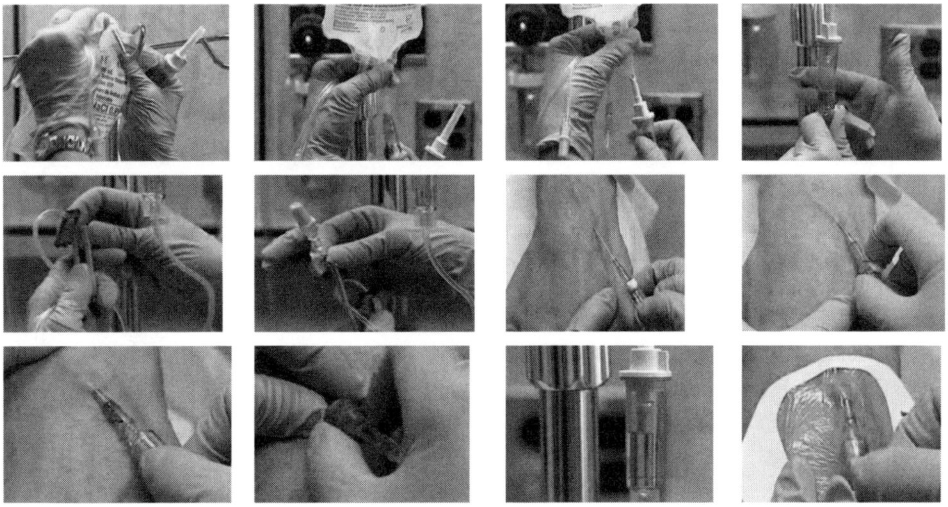

File 4
SELF-ADMINISTERED INJECTIONS

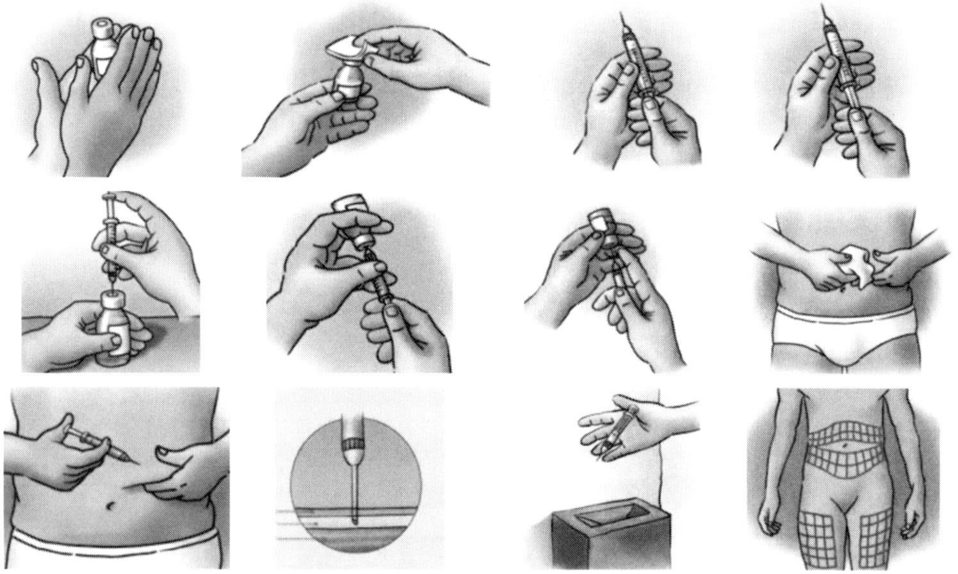

File 5
CHANGING A DRESSING

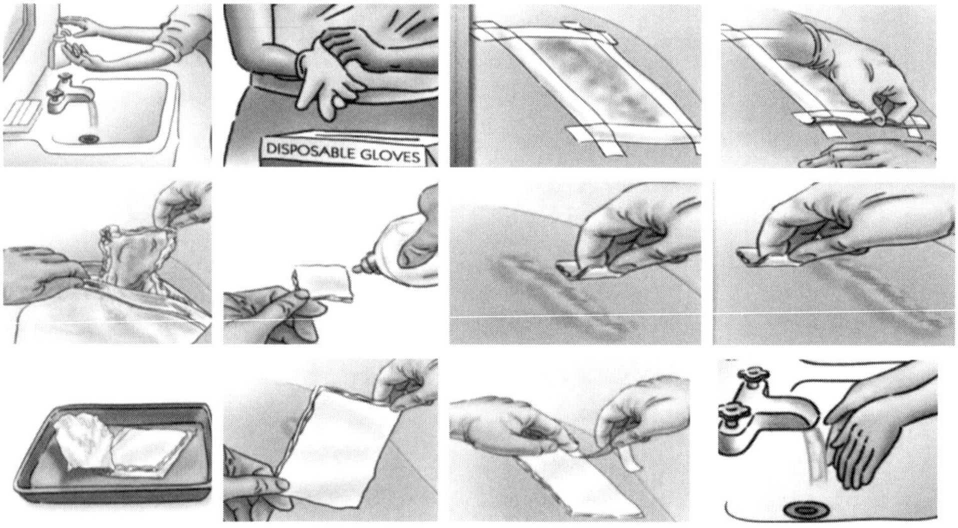

File 6
TAKING A PATIENT'S BLOOD PRESSURE

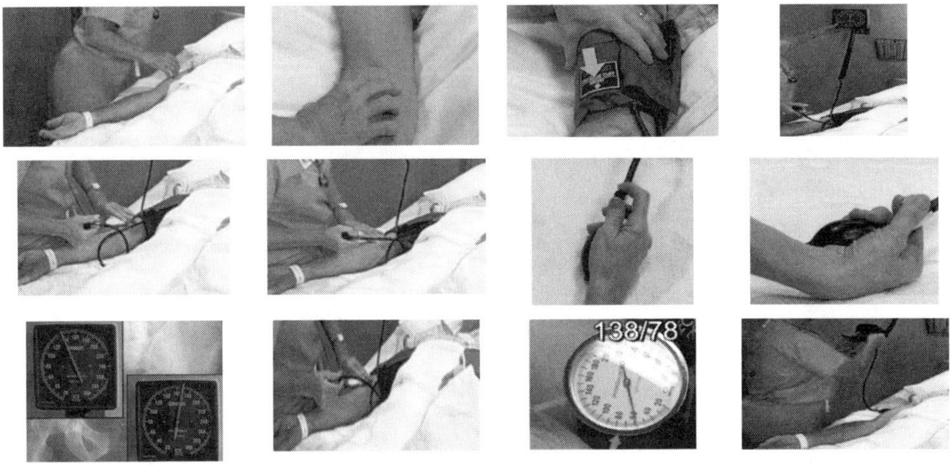

File 7
HAND-WASHING

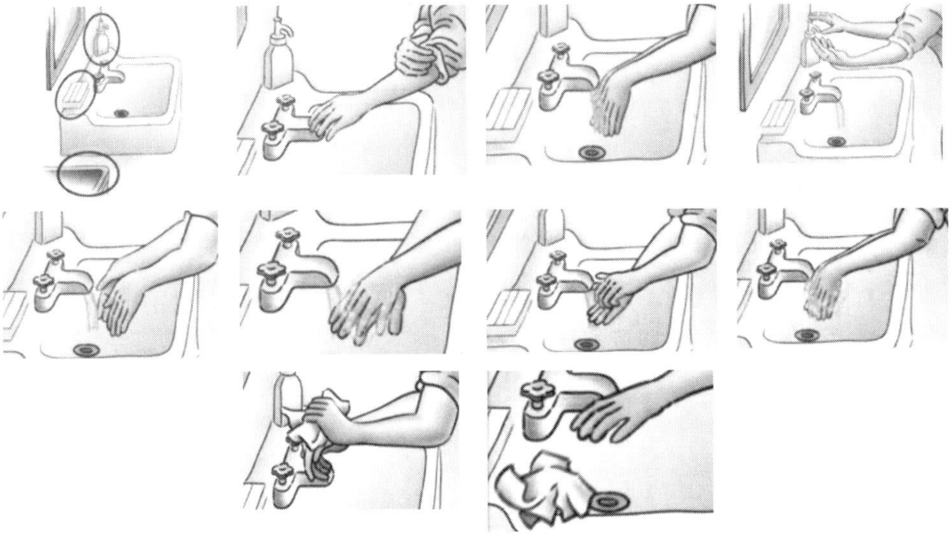

File 8
TAKING A BLOOD SAMPLE

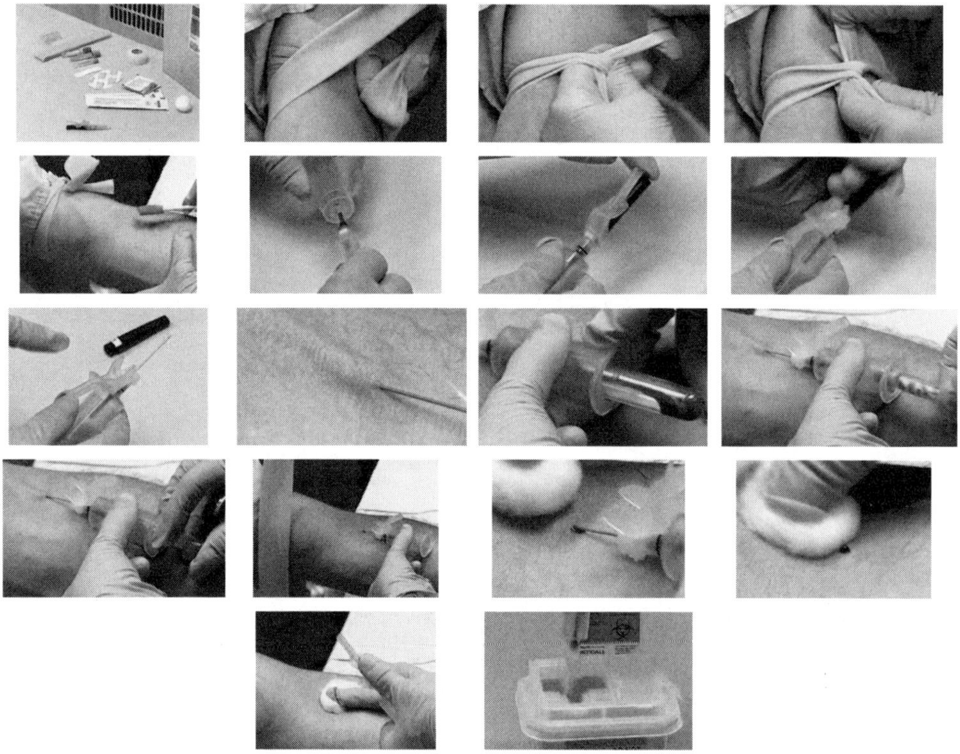

File 9
ASSISTING WITH A BATH

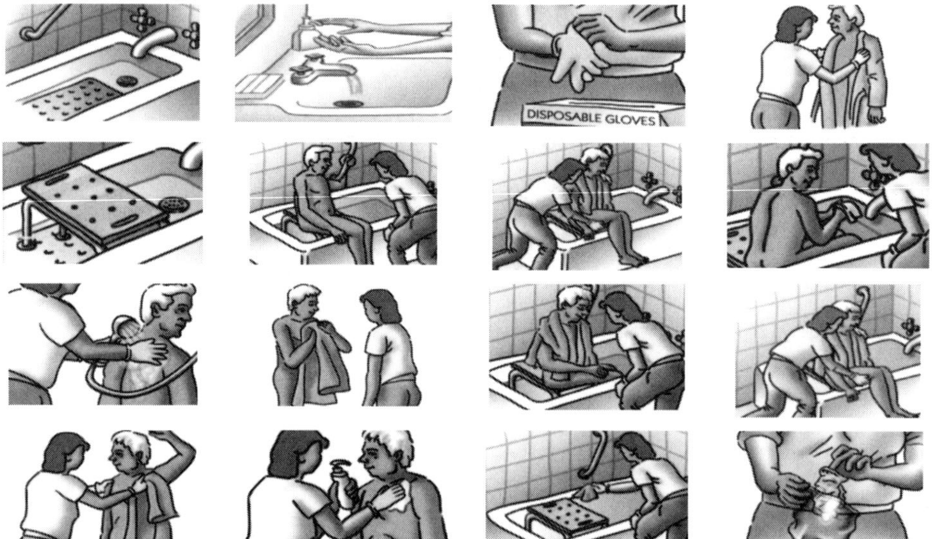

File 10
HELPING THE PATIENT GET OUT OF BED AFTER SURGERY

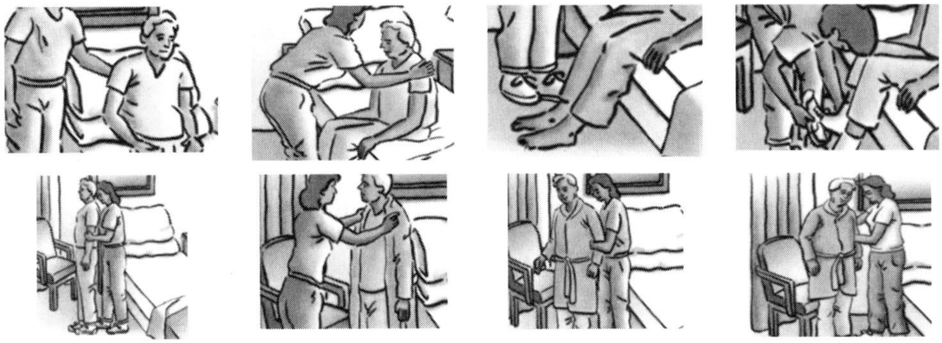

File 11

	a	b	c	d	e	f	g	h	i	j	k	l	m	n	o	p	q	r	s
1	B	R	E	A	S	T	-	F	E	E	D	I	N	G					
2																	M		
3							E	N	T				I				O		D
4													S				O		I
5													O				D		S
6							S	I	T				L			S	S		E
7	R	O	L	L	E	R							A			I			A
8		F	-	I		A		N	E	O	N	A	T	E		B			S
9	E	F	F	E	C	T			A		S		E			L			E
10						E			R							I		S	
11	E															N		T	
12	L		D	R	O	W	S	Y		H	E	A	R	I	N	G		R	R
13	B	M	I												A			O	
14	O														R			N	
15	W				H					S					R		N	G	O
16										U			D		O				
17	B	R	A	I	N			W	I	T	H	D	R	A	W	A	L		
18					G					U			U						
19										R			G		U	N	D	E	R
20										E									

Irregular verbs / Verbes irréguliers

INFINITIF	PRETERIT	PARTICIPE PASSE	TRADUCTION
awake	awoke, awaked	awoken, awaked	(s')éveiller
be	was, were	been	être
bear	bore	borne	porter, supporter
bear	bore	be born	naître
beat	beat	beaten	battre
become	became	become	devenir
begin	began	begun	commencer
bend	bent	bent	courber
bet	bet, betted	bet, betted	parier
bite	bit	bitten	mordre
bleed	bled	bled	saigner
blow	blew	blown	souffler
break	broke	broken	casser
bring	brought	brought	apporter
build	built	built	construire
burn	burnt, burned	burnt, burned	brûler
burst	burst	burst	éclater
buy	bought	bought	acheter
catch	caught	caught	attraper
choose	chose	chosen	choisir
come	came	come	venir
cost	cost	cost	coûter
creep	crept	crept	ramper
cut	cut	cut	couper
deal	dealt	dealt	distribuer
dig	dug	dug	creuser
do	did	done	faire
draw	drew	drawn	tirer, dessiner
dream	dreamt, dreamed	dreamt, dreamed	rêver
drink	drank	drunk	boire
drive	drove	driven	conduire
eat	ate	eaten	manger
fall	fell	fallen	tomber
feed	fed	fed	nourrir
feel	felt	felt	sentir
fly	flew	flown	voler
forbid	forbade, forbad	forbidden	interdire
forget	forgot	forgotten	oublier
forgive	forgave	forgiven	pardonner
freeze	froze	frozen	geler
get	got	got, gotten	obtenir, devenir
give	gave	given	donner
go	went	gone	aller
grow	grew	grown	croître, devenir
hang	hung	hung	pendre
have	had	had	avoir
hear	heard	heard	entendre

INFINITIF	PRETERIT	PARTICIPE PASSE	TRADUCTION
hide	hid	hidden	cacher
hit	hit	hit	frapper
hold	held	held	tenir
hurt	hurt	hurt	blesser, faire mal
keep	kept	kept	garder, conserver
kneel	knelt, kneeled	knelt, kneeled	s'agenouiller
know	knew	known	connaître, savoir
lay	laid	laid	poser
lead	led	led	mener, conduire
lean	leant, leaned	leant, leaned	pencher
learn	learnt, learned	learnt, learned	apprendre
leave	left	left	quitter, laisser
lend	lent	lent	prêter
let	let	let	laisser (faire), louer
lie	lay	lain	être couché
light	lit, lighted	lit, lighted	allumer, éclairer
lose	lost	lost	perdre
make	made	made	faire, fabriquer
mean	meant	meant	signifier, vouloir dire
meet	met	met	rencontrer
mistake	mistook	mistaken	prendre par erreur
overcome	overcame	overcome	surmonter
overtake	overtook	overtaken	dépasser
pay	paid	paid	payer
put	put	put	poser, mettre
quit	quit, quitted	quit, quitted	abandonner, arrêter
read	read	read	lire
ride	rode	ridden	monter (cheval / vélo)
ring	rang	rung	sonner
rise	rose	risen	se lever
run	run	run	courir
saw	sawed	sawn, sawed	scier
say	said	said	dire
see	saw	seen	voir
seek	sought	sought	chercher
sell	sold	sold	vendre
send	sent	sent	envoyer
set	set	set	placer
shake	shook	shaken	secouer, trembler
shine	shone	shone	briller
shoot	shot	shot	tirer, abattre
show	showed	shown, showed	montrer
shut	shut	shut	fermer
sing	sang	sung	chanter
sink	sank	sunk	sombrer, couler
sit	sat	sat	être assis
sleep	slept	slept	dormir
slide	slid	slid	glisser
smell	smelt	smelt	sentir (odorat)
speak	spoke	spoken	parler
spell	spelt, spelled	spelt, spelled	épeler, orthographier

INFINITIF	PRETERIT	PARTICIPE PASSE	TRADUCTION
spend	spent	spent	passer, dépenser
spit	spat	spat	cracher
split	split	split	fendre
spoil	spoilt, spoiled	spoilt, spoiled	gâter
spread	spread	spread	répandre
spring	sprang	sprung	s'élancer
stand	stood	stood	être debout
steal	stole	stolen	voler
stick	stuck	stuck	coller, coincer
stink	stank	stunk	puer
strike	struck	struck	frapper
swear	swore	sworn	jurer
sweep	swept	swept	balayer
swell	swelled	swelled, swollen	enfler
swim	swam	swum	nager
swing	swung	swung	se balancer
take	took	taken	prendre
teach	taught	taught	enseigner
tell	told	told	dire, raconter
think	thought	thought	penser
throw	threw	thrown	jeter
undergo	underwent	undergone	subir
understand	understood	understood	comprendre
undertake	undertook	undertaken	entreprendre
wake	woke	woken	(s')éveiller
wear	wore	worn	porter (vêtements)
weep	wept	wept	pleurer
win	won	won	gagner
wind	wound	wound	enrouler
withdraw	withdrew	withdrawn	retirer
write	wrote	written	écrire

Collocations / Collocations

account for the different factors	prendre en compte les différents facteurs
associated with a low risk	associé à un faible risque
benefit from appropriate treatment	bénéficier d'un traitement adapté
bring on chest pains	déclencher des douleurs thoraciques
care for a patient	soigner / s'occuper d'un patient
consist in administering	consiste à administrer
cope with deadly diseases	faire face à des maladies mortelles
damage to the heart	lésion du coeur
depend on foreign aid	dépendre de l'aide internationale
die from an infection	mourir d'une infection
different from the previous one	différent du précédent
differentiate into rod cells	se différencier en bâtonnets
drop in the death rate	baisse du taux de mortalité
end up with cirrhosis	finir par avoir une cirrhose
excuse me **for** being late	excusez-moi pour mon retard
fall in temperature	baisse de la température
feel like living	avoir envie de vivre
find out what happened	découvrir ce qui s'est passé
improvement in your health	amélioration de votre santé
increase in risk	augmentation des risques
interested in geriatrics	intéressé par la gériatrie
interfere with the production of insulin	entraver la production d'insuline
interspersed with remission periods	entrecoupé de périodes de rémission
involved in a charity	impliqué dans une association caritative
laden with plaques	envahi / surchargé de plaques
look forward to seeing somebody again	avoir hâte de revoir quelqu'un
need for a low-cost vaccine	la nécessité d'un vaccin à bas prix
operate on a patient	opérer un patient
present with signs of hypotonia	présenter des signes d'hypotonie
prevent from developing	empêcher le développement
prior to our research	avant nos travaux de recherche

prone to osteoporosis	sujet à l'ostéoporose
provide with oxygen	fournir de l'oxygène
reduced by 10%	diminué de 10%
referred to as an embolic stroke	dénommé embolie cérébrale
regarded as a preliminary study	considérée comme une étude préliminaire
regardless of age	quel que soit leur âge
rely on a report	s'appuyer sur un rapport
responsible for weight gain	responsable d'une prise de poids
result from brain disorder	être la conséquence de troubles cérébraux
result in grey hair	entraîner l'apparition de cheveux gris
rid the world **of** this plague	débarrasser le monde de ce fléau
screen for prostate cancer	dépister le cancer de la prostate
search for causes	rechercher les causes
sensitivity to light	sensibilité à la lumière
stand for freedom	symboliser la liberté
stem from research	provenir de la recherche
struggle with weight	s'efforcer de perdre du poids
suffer from AMD	souffrir de DMLA
take up smoking	se mettre à fumer
test for HIV	dépister le virus VIH
detrimental to health	nuisible à la santé

GLOSSARY / GLOSSAIRE

A

abdomen	4	abdomen
ability	11	capacité
about	13	environ
academic year	30	année universitaire
accident and emergency department (A&E)	2	les urgences
accompaniment	27	accompagnement
according to	10	selon
accountable	30	responsable
achieve (to)	17	réaliser / accomplir
across from	2	de l'autre côté de
activities of daily living(ADL)	22	activités de la vie quotidienne
actually	11	effectivement / en fait
acute	9	aigüe
acute respiratory distress syndrome (ARDS)	28	syndrome de détresse respiratoire de l'adulte (SDRA)
adaptable	30	souple / qui sait s'adapter
add (to)	18	ajouter
adherence	25	observance / adhérence
adhesive remover	18	dissolvant à colle
adjuvant therapy	29	thérapie adjuvante
administer drugs (to)	25	administrer des médicaments
admissions desk	3	bureau des entrées
admission form	3	formulaire d'entrée
admission reason	3	raison de l'hospitalisation
admitted to hospital (to be)	27	entrer / être admis à l'hôpital
advanced cardiac life support (ACLS)	28	maintien artificiel amélioré des fonctions cardiaques
adverse effects	17	effets indésirables
advice	25	conseil(s)
advise (to)	3	informer / conseiller
advocate (for) (to)	19	préconiser
against the odds	30	contre les aléas
aggressive life-sustaining therapy	27	acharnement thérapeutique
aging	22	vieillissement
agree (to)	19	être d'accord
agreement	11	accord
aim to (to)	8	viser à / avoir pour objectif
airborne infection	20	infection d'origine aérienne
air sac	13	alvéole / sac aérien
alcohol-based hand rub	20	solution hydro-alcoolique pour les mains
alike	25	semblable / similaire
alive	9	en vie
alleviate (to)	10	soulager
allow (to)	10	permettre
along the way	27	au cours de (la maladie…)
along with	12	ainsi que / accompagné de
alveolus (pl. alveoli)	13	alvéole
amazing	11	stupéfiant
ammonia	20	ammoniaque
amount	8	quantité
anaemia	21	anémie
anaesthesia	23	anesthésie
anaesthesiologist (US)	23	anesthésiste

anaesthetic	9	anesthésiant
anaesthetist (GB)	23	anesthésiste
analgesics	10	analgésique
and the like	7	et autres
angina	19	angine de poitrine / angor
ankle	4	cheville
anorexia nervosa	26	anorexie mentale
antidepressant	26	antidépresseur
anus	14	anus
anyway	8	quoi qu'il en soit
aorta	9	aorte
aortic dissection	19	dissection aortique
apart (feet)	23	écartés (pieds)
applicant	30	candidat
apply (to)	18	faire (un pansement) / appliquer
apply for (to)	30	faire une demande / poser sa candidature
apply pressure (to)	16	exercer une pression
arch of aorta	9	crosse de l'aorte
area	11	aire / surface
area	28	domaine
arise (from) (to)	26	provenir (de) / survenir
arm	4	bras
arm	23	accoudoir
armchair	7	fauteuil
around the clock	30	24 heures sur 24
arrhythmia	19	arythmie
arterial blood	16	sang artériel
arterial blood gases (ABG)	28	gaz du sang artériel
arterial oxygen saturation (SaO2)	28	saturation du sang artériel en oxygène
ascending aorta	9	aorte descendante
assess (to)	1	évaluer
assessing pain	8	évaluation de la douleur
assessment	2	évaluation
assign to (to)	2	affecter à
assist (to)	15	aider
at hand	30	à proximité / à disposition
at least	7	au moins
at rest	4	au repos
at the far end	2	au fond de
atherosclerosis	19	athérosclérose
atrial fibrillation	19	fibrillation auriculaire
atrium / atria	9	oreillette
attention deficit hyperactivity disorder (ADHD)	26	trouble d'hyperactivité avec déficit de l'attention (THADA)
autoclave	12	boîte de stérilisation
auxiliary nurse (US)	1	aide-soignante
AV block	19	bloc auriculo-ventriculaire
available	22	disponible
average	22	moyen
avoid (to)	11	éviter
awake	5	éveillé
aware	14	conscient
awareness	19	conscience

B

back and forth	23	d'avant en arrière
backbone	6	colonne vertébrale
bacteria (sg. bacterium)	15	bactéries
balance	11	équilibre
balance (to)	10	équilibrer
band	13	anneau
bandage up (to)	6	bander / mettre un bandage
barefoot	9	nu-pieds
barrel (of a syringe)	17	corps (d'une seringue)
basement	2	sous-sol
basic cardiac life support (BCLS)	28	maintien artificiel des fonctions cardiaques
basically	28	au fond / en fait
bath	22	bain
bath blanket	18	alèse
be called upon (to)	1	être sollicité
be expected to (to)	8	être censé
be in pain (to)	27	souffrir
be willing to (to)	1	être prêt à
bear (to)	8	supporter / tolérer
beat (to)	11	battre
become infected (to)	18	s'infecter
bed linen	18	literie
bedpan	14	bassin hygiénique
bedridden	15	alité / grabataire
bedside table	7	table de chevet
bedsore	18	escarre
bedtime (at)	25	au coucher
behave (to)	21	se comporter
behavioural	19	comportemental
behind	2	derrière
belongings	7	effets personnels
below	6	en dessous
benign	29	bénin
between	2	entre
between jobs	6	en recherche d'emploi
biased (to be)	11	manquer d'objectivité
bin	20	poubelle
binder	18	bandage abdominal
biohazard bag	18	sac biohazard
biopsy	29	biopsie
birth weight (BW)	24	poids de naissance
bits and pieces	7	petites affaires
bladder	15	vessie
blade	23	lame
blanket	7	couverture
bleach	20	eau de javel
bleed back	16	retour veineux
bleeding	9	hémorragie /saignement
blindness	19	cécité
blisters	3	cloques / phlyctènes
blood	11	sang
blood alcohol level (BAL)	21	taux d'alcoolémie
blood bag	21	poche de sang
blood bank	21	banque du sang

blood culture	16	hémoculture
blood donation	21	don du sang
blood electrolytes	16	ionogramme sanguin
blood gases	21	gaz du sang
blood group	21	groupe sanguin
blood pressure (BP)	1	tension artérielle (TA)
blood pressure gauge	12	tensiomètre
blood sugar	14	glycémie
blood test	21	prise de sang
blood transfusion	21	transfusion sanguine
blood tube	21	tube (de prélèvement)
blood typing	21	détermination du groupe sanguin
blood unit	21	unité de sang
blood urea nitrogen (BUN)	21	urée sanguine
bloodstream	20	circulation sanguine
bloodstream infection	20	bactériémie
blood sugar	17	glycémie
bloody (urine)	15	sang (dans les urines)
blow (to)	13	souffler
blunted	26	émoussé
boiling	3	bouillant
bold	22	audacieux / courageux
bone	6	os
bone marrow	16	moelle osseuse
both	26	les deux
bottle	14	pistolet
bottom	11	partie inférieure / bas
bowel	14	intestin
bowel habits	14	habitudes intestinales
bowel movement	14	mouvement intestinal / défécation
box	27	case
BP / blood pressure	1	TA / tension artérielle
bradycardia	19	bradycardie
brain	10	cerveau
brain stem	11	tronc cérébral
break up (to)	14	décomposer
breastbone	6	sternum
breast-feed (to)	26	allaiter
breath	8	respiration
breathe (to)	6	respirer
breathe in (to)	11	inspirer
breathe out (to)	11	expirer
breathing	13	respiration
bring up (to)	5	cracher
broad range of	27	large éventail de
broken line	2	ligne discontinue
bronchiole	13	bronchiole
bronchitis	25	bronchite
bronchus (pl. bronchi)	13	bronche
brother	11	frère
bruise	4	ecchymose / contusion
brush	7	brosse
bug	20	germe / microbe
bulb	19	poire
bulimia nervosa	26	boulimie nerveuse
burning	9	sensation de brûlure
burnout	26	surmenage / épuisement
butterfly stitches	18	steri-strip ®
by the sounds of things	9	d'après ce que vous en dîtes
by the way	10	d'ailleurs / à ce sujet

C

calcaneus / calcaneum	6	calcanéum
calf (pl. calves)	4	mollet
calf bone	6	péroné
call button	3	sonnette
cancel (to)	30	annuler
cap	12	bouchon / capuchon
capillary	14	capillaire
capsule	25	gélule
cardiac arrest	19	arrêt cardiaque
cardiopulmonary resuscitation (CPR)	24	réanimation cardio-pulmonaire (RCP)
cardiovascular system	9	système cardiovasculaire
care	1	soins
care for (to)	24	prendre soin de
carefully	8	attentivement / soigneusement
caregiver (US)	7	accompagnant / aidant
carer (GB)	30	accompagnant / aidant
caring	1	attentionné
carry (to)	10	porter
carry out (to)	8	pratiquer / réaliser
cart (US)	23	chariot (à instruments chirurgicaux)
CAT scan	29	scanner
cath lab = catheterization lab	9	laboratoire de cathétérisme
cause (to)	26	provoquer
ceiling lift	7	lève-malade
cell	14	cellule
cell phone	3	téléphone portable
central nervous system (CNS)	24	système nerveux central
cerebellum	11	cervelet
cerebrospinal fluid (CSF)	24	liquide céphalorachidien
cervix	15	col de l'utérus
challenging situation	30	situation difficile à surmonter
channel	7	chaîne (de télévision)
check (on somebody) (to)	30	vérifier (que quelqu'un va bien)
check out (to)	6	vérifier / examiner
cheek bone	6	pommettes
cheeks	8	joues
chest	4	poitrine / thorax
chew (to)	14	mâcher / mastiquer
children's hospital	2	hôpital d'enfants
chills	5	frissons
chin	8	menton
chlorine	20	chlore
cholesterol blood test	21	test de dépistage du cholestérol
chosen	17	choisi
chronic	9	chronique
chronic obstructive pulmonary disease (COPD)	28	bronchopneumopathie chronique obstructive (BPCO)
cilia	13	cils
circulating nurse	1	infirmière de bloc
clamp	12	pince
clavicle	6	clavicule
cleanse (to)	18	nettoyer
cleansing solution	18	solution de rinçage (de plaie)
clear away (to)	16	dissoudre / éliminer
clogged up	9	obstrué / bouché

close	28	proche
close to	2	près de
closely	28	étroitement / de près
closure	23	fermeture
clot	16	caillot
clothing	19	vêtements
clotting time	16	temps de coagulation
cloudy	15	trouble
cluster	13	amas
coat (to)	13	tapisser
coin (to)	26	inventer / créer
cold	25	rhume
collapse (to)	13	s'affaisser
collarbone	6	clavicule
college	23	institut universitaire
colon	14	côlon
comb	7	peigne
come on (to)	9	survenir
commit to (to)	10	s'engager à
commitment	30	engagement
common	10	fréquent
community nurse (GB)	1	infirmière à domicile / infirmière libérale
companionship	30	réconfort / camaraderie
compatibility	21	compatibilité
complain about / of (to)	15	se plaindre de
complete (to)	7	terminer
complete blood count (CBC) (US)	16	numération formule sanguine (NFS)
complexion	24	teint
compliance	25	observance / adhérence
component	24	paramètre / composant
comprise (to)	30	comprendre
concern	21	inquiétude / crainte
condition	26	état / maladie
confident	30	confiant
consistency	29	régulièrement
consumables	12	produits (de consommation courante)
constricted	9	comprimé
constrictive	9	constrictive
contact person	3	personne à prévenir
continence care	30	soins de la continence
cope with (to)	27	faire face à
cord blood	21	sang de cordon
cornerstone	7	pierre angulaire
coronary artery	9	artère coronaire
coronary artery bypass graft (CABG)	19	pontage coronarien
coronary disease	19	maladie coronarienne
corridor	2	couloir
cotton wool	12	coton hydrophile
cough	5	toux
cough (to)	20	tousser
cough suppressant	25	antitussif
counselling	27	soutien psychologique
countless	1	innombrable
country of origin	3	pays d'origine
course of treatment	27	traitement
coverage	30	couverture (médiatique)
cranium	6	crâne
critical	29	crucial / clé
critically ill	27	gravement malade
crushing	9	sensation d'écrasement

crust	18	croûte
cry (to)	8	pleurer
cubicle	12	box
cuff	19	brassard
culture dish	20	boîte de culture
cup	7	tasse
cupboard	7	placard
cure	17	guérison
cure (to)	11	guérir
curtain	7	rideau
customize (to)	27	personnaliser
cut down on (to)	7	réduire

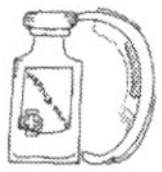

daily	27	quotidien
daily record chart	13	feuille de suivi
damage	10	dégâts
damage (to)	29	endommager
dangle (to)	23	pendre
dare (to)	3	oser
data (pl)	20	données
date of birth (DOB)	3	date de naissance
daughter	11	fille
day procedure unit	2	soins ambulatoires
deal with (to)	8	gérer / maîtriser
death	9	mort
debridement	18	débridement / mise à plat
decade	21	décennie
deep	4	profond
deflate (to)	19	dégonfler
deflect (to)	19	dévier / infléchir
delayed	25	à retardement / différé
delivery	2	accouchement
delivery of care	30	voie d'administration
delivery route	30	administration des soins
delusion	26	délire
demanding	1	exigeant
department	1	service
dermatology	2	dermatologie
descending aorta	9	aorte descendante
design (to)	12	concevoir
desperately	30	terriblement / désespérément
device	9	dispositif / appareil
diabetes blood test	21	test de dépistage du diabète
diaphragm	13	diaphragme
diarrhoea	25	diarrhée
die (to)	9	mourir
diet habits	1	habitudes alimentaires
disabilities	30	handicap
discard (to)	17	jeter
discharge	17	sortie (de l'hôpital)
discomfort	7	(sensation de) gêne
disease	1	maladie

disease-free survival	29	survie sans maladie
disinfect (to)	17	désinfecter
disorder	24	maladie / trouble
display (to)	26	présenter
disposable	17	jetable
disposal	12	élimination
disposal bag	18	sac à déchets
dispose of (to)	12	jeter
district nurse (GB)	1	infirmière à domicile / infirmière libérale
divorced	3	divorcé(e)
dizziness	15	vertiges / étourdissements
do the job (to)	15	faire l'affaire
DOB / date of birth	3	date de naissance
document (to)	18	noter / enregistrer
don (to)	23	enfiler
donate (to)	11	donner
donation	11	don
donor	11	donneur
doorbell	28	sonnette
dosage	5	posologie
drainage	18	écoulement
drapes	18	champ stérile
draw away (to)	15	aspirer
draw blood (to)	21	prélever du sang
drawer	7	tiroir
dress (a wound) (to)	4	panser (une plaie)
dress (to)	22	habiller
dressing	4	pansement
dressing gown	7	robe de chambre
drip chamber	16	chambre compte-goutte
drop in	17	chute
drowsy	24	somnolent
drug	25	médicament
drug delivery	30	administration des médicaments
dry (to)	18	sécher / assécher
dry (cough)	25	(toux) sèche
dull	9	sourde
dull (to)	10	atténuer
dummy	11	mannequin
duodenum	14	duodénum
duties	1	tâches

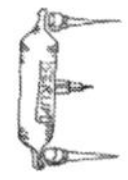

ears	8	oreilles
earth (the)	6	la terre
ease (to)	10	calmer
ECG (GB) / EKG (US)	9	ECG
edges (of a wound)	16	bords / lèvres (d'une plaie)
e.g. / exempli gratia	12	par exemple
effective	26	efficace
efficacy	27	efficacité
elbow	4	coude
elderly	14	âgé / personnes âgées
electrolytes	14	ionogramme

elevator (US)	2	ascenseur
eligible	21	répondant aux critères
emergency room (ER)	1	les urgences
enable (to)	30	permettre
end	13	extrémité
end of life	27	fin de vie
end-of-life care	30	soins de fin de vie
end up in (to)	27	finir à
endotracheal tube (ET)	28	sonde d'intubation
enlarged	25	hypertrophié
enough	22	assez / suffisamment
enteral feeding	28	alimentation entérale
epidemic	19	épidémie
epiglottis	14	épiglotte
erythrocyte sedimentation rate (ESR)	16	vitesse de sédimentation (VS)
escape (to)	19	échapper
euthanasia	27	euthanasie
even	10	même
event	26	événement
eventually	8	finalement
excruciating	9	atroce
eye drops	25	collyre
eyebrows	8	sourcils
eyelashes	8	cils
eyelids	8	paupières
eyes	8	yeux

F

face mask	23	masque chirurgical
facility	22	établissement
fail (to)	10	échouer / ne pas réussir à
failure	11	insuffisance / défaillance
failure to thrive (FTT)	24	retard de croissance
fairly	9	assez / plutôt
fall	7	chute
fall apart (to)	16	se désagréger
Fallopian tube	15	trompes de Fallope
family doctor	3	médecin généraliste
family name	3	nom de famille
fashion	25	manière
fasten (to)	23	attacher
fasting glucose	21	glycémie à jeun
fearfulness	26	crainte
features	8	traits / caractéristiques
feces	14	matières fécales / excréments
feed (to)	8	alimenter
feeding bag	14	poche d'alimentation
feel like (to)	9	avoir l'impression que
feel sick (to)	25	avoir la nausée
female	3	féminin
femur	6	fémur
fever	25	fièvre
fibula	6	péroné

fight	20	combat
figure	20	chiffre
finger	4	doigt
(finger) nail	20	ongle
fill (to)	13	remplir
find out (to)	12	chercher à savoir
finding	18	résultat / symptôme / découverte
fine	5	bien / en bonne forme
fingertip	20	extrémité du doigt
first floor (GB)	2	premier étage
first name	3	prénom
first of all	8	tout d'abord
first storey (US)	2	rez-de-chaussée
fist	11	poing
fit together (to)	14	s'articuler
fitted with	6	équipé de
flat	21	(à) plat
flex (to)	4	fléchir
floor	2	sol / étage
flow	16	débit / flux
flow (to)	9	circuler / couler
fluid	18	liquide
flush out (to)	15	nettoyer / rincer
focus on (to)	7	se concentrer sur
folks (US)	27	les gens
food intake	22	prise alimentaire
foodborne infection	20	infection d'origine alimentaire
foot (pl. feet)	4	pied
foot(ft)	24	pied (30,48 cm)
forceps	12	forceps
forearm	4	avant-bras
forehead	8	front
foreign	12	étranger
forte	27	point fort
fortunately	27	heureusement
foul-smelling	18	nauséabond
fracture and pain clinic	2	service d'orthopédie et de traumatologie / unité d'évaluation et de traitement de la douleur
frail	22	frêle / fragile
framework of bones	6	structure osseuse
friendliness	22	gentillesse
frightening	9	effrayant
frontline	20	première ligne / front
full	16	plein
full blood count (FBC) (GB)	16	numération formule sanguine (NFS)
full term (FT)	24	né à terme
full term normal delivery (FTND)	24	accouchement à terme normal
fund (to)	28	financer
funding	30	financement
fungal infection	20	mycose
fungus (pl fungi)	20	champignon
funny bone	6	humérus
further	30	complémentaire / supplémentaire

G

gallbladder	14	vésicule biliaire
gasp for air (to)	9	suffoquer / haleter
gastro-intestinal system	14	système digestif
gate 1	2	porte 1
gather (to)	13	récupérer / rassembler
gauze	12	gaze
gender	3	sexe
general practitioner (GP)	3	médecin généraliste (MG)
generalised anxiety disorder	26	troubles de l'angoisse généralisés
genitourinary system	15	système génito-urinaire
gently	15	délicatement / doucement
germ	20	germe
germ-free	23	stérile / aseptisé
get rid of (to)	11	éliminer / se débarrasser de
get used to (to)	8	s'habituer à
gift	11	don / cadeau
given	28	étant donné
given name	3	prénom
gloves	12	gants
glycaemia	21	glycémie
go ahead (to)	18	continuer / reprendre
go straight ahead / on (to)	2	continuer tout droit
go through (to)	11	passer en revue
goal	10	but
god	6	dieu
going on	17	en cours
gown	23	sarrau / blouse
GP	3	médecin généraliste (MG)
grade	21	qualité / type
graduate (to)	23	obtenir un diplôme / une licence
graft	23	greffe / greffon
grape-like	13	en forme de grappe
grateful	8	reconnaissant
graze	4	éraflure
greenish-looking	5	d'aspect verdâtre
grind (to)	14	écraser / broyer
grip	4	force de préhension
ground floor (GB)	2	rez-de-chaussée
grow (to)	20	se développer / proliférer
grow over (to)	16	recouvrir
growing	15	croissant
guided tour	2	visite guidée
guidelines	25	consignes / instructions / recommandations
gut	29	intestin

H

hair	8	cheveux
hairs	8	poils
hand	4	main
hand-held	9	portatif
handle (to)	27	supporter
handover	28	transmission
hands-on approach	19	approche pragmatique
hang (to)	16	pendre / suspendre
hang by a thread (to)	11	tenir à un fil
hardly	8	à peine / guère
harm	25	mal
harmful	25	nocif
harmless	25	inoffensif
head	4	tête
head into (to)	30	se diriger (vers)
head circumference (HC)	24	périmètre de la tête
head nurse (US)	1	infirmière en chef
headache	5	mal de tête / céphalée
heal (to)	4	cicatriser / guérir
healing process	7	guérison
health	10	santé
health care facility	12	établissement de soins de santé
health care provider	15	personnel soignant
health education	30	hygiène publique
health visitor	30	infirmière des services sociaux
healthy	1	en bonne santé
heart	6	cœur
heart attack	9	crise cardiaque
heart disease	19	maladie cardiaque
heart failure	19	insuffisance cardiaque
heart-healthy diet	19	régime alimentaire sain pour le cœur
heart rate	11	fréquence cardiaque
heel bone	6	calcanéum
height (Ht)	24	taille
haemostat	5	hémostat
heel	4	talon
helpline	23	centre d'assistance téléphonique
heroic treatment	27	acharnement thérapeutique
high blood pressure (HBP)	19	hypertension artérielle
hip	4	hanche
history taking	5	interrogatoire
HIV test	21	test de dépistage VIH
hold (to)	13	maintenir
hold accountable (to)	22	tenir responsable de
hold on (to)	30	patienter
hold one's breath (to)	13	retenir sa respiration
hold up (to)	6	soutenir
hole	16	trou
Holy Grail	21	quête ultime / Saint Graal
home	30	maison / foyer
home address	3	adresse personnelle
homebound	30	bloqué à la maison

hospital admission	3	entrée à l'hôpital
hospital stay	29	séjour hospitalier
hospital trust (GB)	20	hôpital public (autonome)
hospital-acquired infection	20	infection hospitalière
housebound	30	bloqué / confiné à la maison
human body	4	corps humain
humerus	6	humérus
hunt around (to)	12	chercher partout
hurt (to)	6	faire mal

ice	30	glace / verglas
ICU nurse	28	infirmière en soins intensifs
icy	30	glacial
ilium	6	ilion
illness	26	maladie
impairment	22	altération / dégradation
implement (to)	19	mettre en œuvre
improve (to)	10	améliorer
improvement	10	amélioration
in front of	2	devant
in labour	2	en travail
in the way (to be)	19	gêner
in vitro fertilization (IVF)	21	fécondation in vitro (FIV)
inability	26	incapacité
inch (in)	24	2,54 cm
increase (to)	19	augmenter
individually-tailored care	30	soins individualisés
induction course	11	stage d'accueil
inexpensive	12	peu coûteux / bon marché
infant	8	nourrisson / bébé
infection	18	infection
inferior vena cava	9	veine cave inférieure
inflate (to)	20	gonfler
influenza / the flu	25	grippe
inhaler	25	inhalateur
inherited	26	génétique / hérité
injection	17	injection / piqûre
injection-free	17	sans piqûre
injure (to)	6	blesser / se faire mal à
injured (the)	1	blessés (les)
injury	7	blessure
inner	13	interne
inoculation	17	inoculation
insulin injection	17	piqûre d'insuline
insulin pen	17	stylo à insuline
intensive care unit (ICU)	2	soins intensifs
interlinked (to be)	11	(être) lié
internal organs	11	organes internes
intertwine (to)	20	(entre)croiser
intra-uterine growth retardation (IUGR)	24	retard de croissance intra-utérin
intravenous line (IV)	3	perfusion / intraveineuse
introduce oneself (to)	2	se présenter

involvement	7	implication
iron deficiency	21	carence en fer
ischium	6	ischion
islet	17	îlot
issue	11	question / numéro
item (of clothing)	28	article (vestimentaire)

J

jab	4	injection / piqûre
joint	6	articulation
journey	16	voyage

K

keep an eye on (to)	8	surveiller
key	19	(élémcnt) clef
keyhole surgery	23	chirurgie endoscopique / cœlioscopie
keypad	2	clavier
kid	30	enfant / gamin
kidney	11	rein
kitchen	14	cuisine
knee	4	genou
kneecap	6	rotule
knock on (to)	2	frapper à
knowledge	23	savoir / connaissance

L

lab(oratory)	17	labo(ratoire)
labour and birthing suite	2	salle de travail et d'accouchement
lacteal	14	chylifère
lancet	23	lancette
large intestine	11	gros intestin
larynx	13	larynx
last name (US)	3	nom de famille
late march (in)	8	fin mars
latest	15	tout dernier
layer	11	membrane / couche
lead (to)	26	mener

lead maternity carer	2	responsable des soins
lead to (to)	2	mener à / conduire à
leadership	30	qualités de chef
leading cause	15	cause principale / première cause
leads	10	dérivations
leaflet	28	brochure / dépliant
leakage	15	fuite
leap	21	avancée considérable / bond en avant
leg	4	jambe
leg ulcer care	30	soins d'ulcères de jambe
legionellosis	20	légionellose
legionnaire's disease	20	maladie du légionnaire
lend (to)	21	prêter
level	17	taux / niveau
level out the playing field (to)	22	mettre sur un pied d'égalité
liability	15	responsabilité civile
licensed practical nurse (LPN)	1	infirmière auxiliaire (Canada)
lie (to)	12	être allongé
life (pl. lives)	9	vie
lifespan	19	durée de vie
lifestyle	19	mode de vie / règles hygiéno-diététiques
life-threatening	27	qui engage le pronostique vital
lift	2	ascenseur
lift (to)	10	soulever
likely to	20	susceptible de
line	16	intraveineuse
linen	2	service de lingerie
lip	8	lèvre
liver	11	foie
lobe	13	lobe
localised	9	locale
locked	2	fermé à clef
locker	7	casier
lock-out interval	17	période réfractaire
long-term disease (LTD)	30	affection de longue durée
long-term illness	30	affection de longue durée
long-term memory	22	mémoire des faits anciens
loop	21	boucle
loose stools	14	selles diarrhéiques / peu consistantes
loosely	6	assez librement / vaguement
loosen (to)	18	ramollir
loss	16	perte
loved one	7	être cher
low birth weight (LBW)	24	faible poids de naissance
low-back pain	10	douleur lombaire
lower airways	13	voies respiratoires inférieures
lower jaw	6	mâchoire inférieure
lower limb	4	membre inférieur
lower oneself (into a chair) (to)	23	se laisser glisser / s'asseoir
lumbar puncture (LP)	24	ponction lombaire
lumpectomy	29	chirurgie mammaire conservatrice
lung	6	poumon
lung function test	13	explorations fonctionnelles respiratoires
lymph node	29	ganglion lymphatique

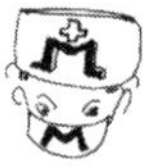

maiden name	3	nom de jeune fille
main entrance	2	entrée principale
make sure (to)	20	vérifier / s'assurer que
make up	7	maquillage
make up (to)	13	former / constituer
male	3	masculin
male nurse	1	infirmier
malignant	29	malin
malodorous	18	malodorant
manage (to)	19	prendre en charge
management	8	prise en charge
mandible	6	mandibule
marital status	3	situation familiale
mark	1	note
married	3	marié(e)
marrow	11	moelle
mat	22	tapis (de bain)
maternity	2	maternité
maxilla	6	maxillaire
meal	2	repas
mean corpuscular volume (MCV)	16	volume glomérulaire moyen (VGM)
means (a)	15	un moyen
meanwhile	13	pendant ce temps
measles, mumps and rubella (MMR)	24	rougeole, oreillons, rubéole (ROR)
mechanical ventilation (MV)	28	ventilation mécanique
medic	17	médecin
medical file	3	dossier médical
medical record	7	dossier médical
medication	3	médicaments / traitement
meet the needs of (to)	27	satisfaire les besoins de
melancholy	26	mélancolie
memory	22	mémoire
memory loss	22	perte de mémoire
metastasis (pl. metastases)	29	métastase
metastasize (to)	29	se métastaser
microwave oven	2	four à micro-ondes
mild	9	discrète
mind	26	esprit
Mini Mental Status Examination	17	test de Folstein
mistake	25	erreur / faute
mitral valve	9	valve mitrale
moan (to)	8	gémir / geindre
moderate	9	moyenne / modérée
moisten (to)	13	humidifier
moisture	15	humidité
moisture proof	18	étanche
monitor (to)	9	surveiller
mood disorder	26	trouble de l'humeur
mood swings	26	sautes d'humeur
mop (to)	22	passer la serpillère
mostly	20	la plupart du temps
motions	14	selles

mouth	8	bouche
mouthpiece	13	embout
MRSA / methicillin-resistant staphylococcus aureus	20	SARM / staphylococcus aureus résistant à la méthicilline
mucosa	14	muqueuse
multiple organ failure (MOF)	28	déficience polyviscérale
muscle bulk	4	volume musculaire
muscle tone	4	tonus musculaire
myocardial infarction (MI)	19	infarctus du myocarde
myocardium	9	myocarde

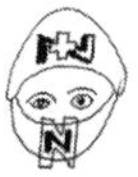

napkin	7	serviette de table
nasal cavity	13	cavité nasale
nasal spray	25	spray nasal
nasty	4	méchant
national health insurance number	3	numéro de sécurité sociale
National Health Service (NHS)	30	branche maladie du régime de sécurité sociale britannique
near	2	près de
nearby	20	à proximité
nearly	25	presque
neck	3	cou
needle	16	aiguille
needle disposal container	17	boîte jette-aiguille
needle guard	21	gaine de protection
needless to say	14	cela va sans dire
needle-stick injury	17	blessure par piqûre d'aiguille
negative pressure ventilation (NPV)	28	ventilation à pression négative
nervous breakdown	26	dépression nerveuse
newborn	24	nouveau né
next of kin	3	parent le plus proche
next to	2	près de
nightmare	25	cauchemar
nitrogen	14	azote
no hard and fast rules	7	pas de règles absolues
no matter what	30	quel que soit
non-disruptive	7	calme / non perturbant
nose	8	nez
nostrils	8	narine
notice (to)	1	remarquer
numb	9	engourdi
nurse	1	infirmière
nurse's aide (GB)	1	aide soignante
nursing	1	soins infirmiers
nursing home	22	maison de retraite médicalisée (EHPAD)
nursing officer	1	cadre de santé
nursing school / school of nursing	1	institut de formation en soins infirmiers (IFSI)
nursing station	2	poste de soins infirmiers
nursing student (US)	1	étudiant infirmier / infirmière
nutrient	14	nutriment

observance	25	observance / adhérence
obsessive compulsive disorder (OCD)	26	trouble obsessionnel compulsif (TOC)
occupation	3	profession
occur (to)	9	survenir / arriver
oesophagus / gullet	14	œsophage
off sick	15	malade / arrêté en congé maladie
ointment	4	pommade
old-age pensioner	11	retraité
on an empty stomach	21	à jeun
on call (room)	2	salle d'astreinte
on the left	2	à gauche
on the other side of	2	de l'autre côté de
on the premises	14	sur place / dans les locaux
on the right	2	à droite
once	9	une fois/ une fois que
once	22	autrefois
oncology nurse	29	infirmière en oncologie
one to one nursing	28	soins individuels
one-size-fits-all approach	27	approche universelle
ongoing	30	continu / suivi
ooze (to)	18	suppurer / suinter
outpatient department (OPD)	2	consultations externes
operate on a patient (to)	23	opérer un patient
operating room (OR)	23	salle d'opération / bloc opératoire
operating table	23	table d'opération
operating theatre (GB)	23	salle d'opération / bloc opératoire
opposite	2	en face de
oral cavity	14	cavité buccale
organ	11	organe
organs at risk (OAR)	29	organes à risque
outcome	28	devenir / issue
outer	15	externe
outlook	26	perspectives
outpatient	29	(en) ambulatoire
ovary	17	ovaire
over	11	terminé
over the counter (OTC)	5	en vente libre
over there	2	là-bas
overactive	25	hyperactif
overall	1	globalement / dans l'ensemble
overcome (to)	21	surmonter
overdose	25	surdosage
overdue	22	attendu depuis longtemps
overlapping	24	qui se recouvre
overnight	7	pour la nuit
override (to)	30	l'emporter sur
override button	2	bouton d'accès direct
overview	1	vue d'ensemble
overweight	19	surpoids / en surpoids
own	26	propre à soi / personnel

P

P / pulse	5	pouls
pack (to)	12	emballer
packed lunch	2	panier-repas
pad	18	tampon / compresse
paediatric nurse	24	infirmière en pédiatrie
pain	8	douleur
pain assessment	10	évaluation de la douleur
pain clinic	10	centre anti-douleur
pain management	10	prise en charge de la douleur
pain relief	10	soulagement de la douleur
painful	6	douloureux
painkiller	5	anti-douleur / analgésique
pal	3	copain / copine / pote
palliative care	27	soins palliatifs
palm	20	paume
pan	15	casserole
pancreas	14	pancréas
panic attacks	26	crise d'angoisse
panic disorder	26	trouble panique
paranoia	26	paranoïa
paranoid	26	paranoïaque
partial pressure of oxygen in arterial blood (PaO2)	28	pression en oxygène dans le sang artériel
pass on (an infection) (to)	20	transmettre (une infection)
pass through (to)	29	traverser
pass urine (to)	25	uriner
pass water (to)	15	uriner
passive stretch	4	étirement passif
patella	6	rotule
patented	15	breveté
patient's chart	15	feuille de suivi
patient's room	7	chambre du patient
peak airflow	13	débit expiratoire de pointe
peak flow meter	13	débitmètre de pointe
peak inspiratory pressure (PIP)	28	pression inspiratoire de pointe (PIP)
peel away (to)	18	décoller / retirer
pelvis	6	bassin
penis	15	pénis
perform (to)	8	pratiquer / réaliser
perform an operation (to)	23	effectuer une opération
pericarditis	19	péricardite
personal details	3	renseignements personnels
personal particulars	3	renseignements personnels
PET scan	29	TEP / PET
petrol	10	essence
pharmacy (US)	2	pharmacie
physical therapy	10	kinésithérapie
physician (US)	27	médecin
physician-assisted suicide	27	suicide médicalement assisté
physiotherapy	2	kinésithérapie
pick up (to)	14	absorber / se saisir de
pill	25	pilule

pillow	7	oreiller
pinched	10	pincé / coincé
plaster	12	sparadrap
platelet	16	plaquette
play it by ear (to)	8	se fier à son instinct
plea	21	appel / plaidoyer
plenty of	3	beaucoup de
pleura	13	plèvre
pleural cavity	13	cavité pleurale
pleural space	13	cavité pleurale
plot (to)	26	comploter
plug	16	bouchon
plug (to)	16	boucher / obstruer
plunger	17	piston
pool	2	baignoire
port / portacath	29	cathéter à chambre implantable
positive end expiratory pressure (PEEP)	28	pression positive en fin d'expiration
positive pressure ventilation (PPV)	28	ventilation à pression positive
post-operative care	23	soins post-opératoires
post-partum psychosis	26	psychose puerpérale
post-traumatic stress disorder (PTSD)	26	état de stress post-traumatique
pound (lb)	24	livre (0,45 kg)
pour (to)	18	verser
powerful	8	puissant
practical nursing skills	1	techniques infirmières
precancerous polyps	29	polypes précancéreux
predicament	11	situation difficile
pregnancy (Pg)	24	grossesse
pregnant (Pg)	24	enceinte
premises (on the)	14	sur place / dans les locaux
prep (to)	16	préparer
prescriber	26	médecin prescripteur
pretty badly	3	assez sévèrement
prevent (to)	7	prévenir / empêcher
prick (to)	12	piquer
primary care	30	soins de première intention / de santé primaire
prior	28	précédent / antérieur
private health insurance	3	assurance complémentaire / mutuelle
probe	12	sonde
procedure	9	intervention
professional address	3	adresse professionnelle
prognosis	29	pronostic
promote (to)	19	promouvoir
proof of principle	21	validation de principe
propel (to)	13	propulser
proper	12	adéquat / correct
properly	10	correctement
prostate	15	prostate
prove (fatal) (to)	17	s'avérer (fatal)
provide (to)	7	fournir
provider	18	médecin soignant
psychiatric nurse	26	infirmière en psychiatrie
psychiatrist	26	psychiatre
psychosis	26	psychose
psychotic	26	psychotique
pull (to)	4	tirer
pulmonary artery	9	artère pulmonaire
pulmonary trunk	9	tronc pulmonaire
pulmonary vein	9	veine pulmonaire
pulse (P)	5	pouls

puncture	21	ponction
purpose	2	but / objectif
purulent	18	purulent
pus	18	pus
push (to)	4	pousser
put on hold (to)	30	mettre en attente
put to sleep (to)	9	endormir
put up with (to)	10	supporter / faire avec

Q

qualified nurse	1	infirmière diplômée
quality of life (QOL)	22	qualité de vie
quite a lot of time	14	pas mal de temps

R

radiating	9	qui irradie
radius	6	radius
raise (to)	21	soulever
randomly assigned	17	répartis de façon aléatoire
range	28	éventail / gamme
range from ... to (to)	1	varier de … à / aller de … à
rate	24	taux / fréquence
rate (to)	22	évaluer
raw number	22	chiffre brut
razor	7	rasoir
reach (to)	3	joindre / atteindre
reading	13	relevé / mesure
recipient (US)	11	receveur
reconstruction surgery	29	chirurgie réparatrice
(medical) record	18	dossier (médical)
record (to)	13	relever / enregistrer
recover (to)	29	se régénérer / se rétablir / récupérer
recovery	17	guérison
recovery room	23	salle de réveil
rectum	14	rectum
red blood cell (RBC)	16	globule rouge
redundancies	5	licenciements
refer (to)	29	faire référence à
referral	27	transfert / orientation (du patient)
referring doctor	3	médecin référent
rehabilitation ward	2	unité de rééducation
relapse	29	récidive
relapse-free survival	29	survie sans récidive
relationship with the patient	3	lien de parenté avec le patient
relative	3	parent

release (to)	19	dévisser / ouvrir / libérer
relentless	20	acharné / sans merci
relevant	30	pertinent
reliable	30	fiable
reliance	15	dépendance
relief	8	soulagement
relieve (to)	10	soulager
relocation	5	délocalisation
remain (to)	8	rester
remission	29	rémission
remote device	10	télécommande
removal	12	élimination
remove (to)	4	retirer / dégager / procéder à l'ablation
renal failure (RF)	28	insuffisance rénale
replenish (to)	16	remplacer
require (to)	3	nécessiter / exiger
reschedule (to)	30	reprogrammer
residential care home	30	foyer / logement pour personnes âgées
resourceful	30	plein de ressources / ingénieux
respiratory distress	13	détresse respiratoire
respiratory distress syndrome (RDS)	28	syndrome de détresse respiratoire
respiratory rate (RR)	24	fréquence respiratoire
respiratory system	13	système respiratoire
respond to treatment (to)	29	répondre au traitement
responsive	20	réactif / sensible à
rest	29	repos
restaurant	2	restaurant
restful	25	réparateur / paisible
restlessness	26	agitation
restroom (US)	3	toilettes / WC
retain (to)	23	oublier / laisser
rewarding	1	gratifiant / enrichissant
rib	6	côte
right	9	bon / juste
right away	10	immédiatement
right in the middle	9	en plein milieu
ringing in the ears	25	bourdonnements d'oreilles
risk factor	19	facteur de risque
robe	23	robe de chambre
roller clamp	16	molette
root	10	racine
(doctor's) round	28	visite (au chevet du malade)
route of administration	30	voie d'administration
row	13	rangée
RR / respiratory rate	24	fréquence respiratoire
rub (to)	20	frotter
run (to)	25	gérer / diriger
run out of (to)	16	être à court de
runny nose	24	nez qui coule
rush (to)	9	précipiter

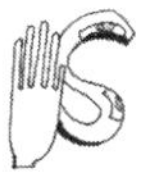

(state) registered nurse (SRN) / (RN)	1	infirmière diplômée d'Etat (IDE)
sacrum	6	sacrum
safe	1	sûr / sans danger
safety	1	sécurité
safety check	5	précaution
salivary gland	14	glande salivaire
sanitize (to)	12	assainir / aseptiser
save (to)	9	gagner / économiser
scab	18	croûte
scald oneself (to)	3	s'ébouillanter
scale	8	échelle
scale up (to)	21	passer à l'échelle / à la vitesse supérieure
scalp	3	cuir chevelu
scalpel	12	scalpel
scapula	6	omoplate
scar	18	cicatrice
scarring	18	cicatrisation
scary	9	effrayant / terrifiant
scientist	21	chercheur
scissors	12	ciseaux
screen (to)	18	dépister / repérer
screw (to)	16	visser
scrotum	15	scrotum
scrub (to)	23	laver / désinfecter
scrub nurse (US)	1	instrumentiste / panseuse
scrubbing	23	lavage chirurgical des mains
seal off (to)	14	obstruer
sealed	14	sur place
search for (to)	10	chercher
second storey (US)	2	premier étage
secure (to)	18	fixer
seek (to)	19	(re)chercher
seizure	24	crise (épileptique)
self-esteem	26	estime de soi / amour propre
self-inflicted wound	26	automutilation
self-renewing	21	auto-régénérant
semester	1	semestre
sensitive	14	sensible
serious (illness)	27	(maladie) grave
session	10	séance
set	12	ensemble
set the stage (to)	15	planter le décor
set up (to)	16	mettre en place
set up an I.V. (to)	16	mettre en place une perfusion
setting	12	cadre / contexte / environnement
settle in (to)	7	s'installer
sexually-transmitted disease (STD)	24	maladie sexuellement transmissible (MST)
sexually-transmitted diseases blood test	21	test de dépistage MST
sexually-transmitted infection (STI)	24	infection sexuellement transmissible (IST)
shaking	25	tremblement
shallow	8	peu profond
shallow angle	21	angle relativement faible

shape	6	forme
share (to)	7	partager
sharp	9	vif / intense
sharp end	17	extrémité pointue
shaving foam	7	mousse à raser
sheet	7	drap
(information) sheet	26	plaquette (d'information)
shift	28	équipe
shin bone	6	tibia
shooting (pain)	9	(douleur) lancinante
short of breath	27	essoufflé
shortage	15	pénurie
short-term memory	22	mémoire des faits récents
shot	17	injection / piqûre
shoulder	4	épaule
shoulder blade	6	omoplate
shoulder girdle	6	ceinture scapulaire
shower	2	douche
sibling	26	frère ou sœur
sick	25	nauséeux / malade
sick (the)	1	malades (les)
side-effects	17	effets secondaires
significantly	10	de manière significative
since	1	puisque
single	3	célibataire
single	29	unique / seul
sink	23	évier
sister	1	infirmière en chef
sit up (to)	23	s'asseoir bien droit
size	11	taille
skeletal system	6	système squelettique
skeleton	6	squelette
skilled	29	compétent / qualifié
skills	1	compétences
skin	16	peau
skin breakdown	22	lésion cutanée
skull	6	crâne
sleet	30	grésil
sleeve	20	manche
slice	11	tranche
slightly	10	légèrement
slip (to)	15	glisser
slipped disc	10	hernie discale
slippers	23	pantoufles
slow down (to)	8	ralentir
small intestine	11	intestin grêle
smelly	15	malodorant
smile (to)	8	sourire
smoothly	4	sans à-coups / en douceur
sneeze (to)	20	éternuer
snow	30	neige
soap	7	savon
soap dispenser	20	distributeur de savon
social phobia	26	phobie sociale
soft tissues	6	tissus mous
soil	12	terre / souillures
soil (to)	12	souiller
solely	28	uniquement
son	11	fils
sooner	9	plus tôt

soothe (to)	10	calmer
sound (to)	21	paraître
speech and language therapy	2	orthophonie
spend (time) (to)	14	passer (du temps)
spermatic cord	15	cordon spermatique
spike	16	perforateur
spill	15	flaque
spinal column	6	colonne vertébrale
spinal cord	10	moelle épinière
spine	6	colonne vertébrale
spleen	11	rate
sponge	6	éponge
spongy	11	spongieux
sprain (to)	6	faire une entorse
spread (to)	4	écarter / se propager
spread to (to)	20	se transmettre à
sputum	5	expectoration
square meter	13	mètre carré
squeeze (to)	4	serrer
stabbing	9	en coup de poignard
stack	6	empilement
staff	1	le personnel
staff canteen	2	cantine / cafétéria du personnel
staff nurse	1	infirmière hospitalière
stage	29	stade
stairs	2	escaliers
stand for (to)	15	signifier / vouloir dire
stand out (to)	22	se distinguer
stand still (to)	23	se tenir immobile
staple	12	agrafe
state (to)	5	indiquer
state registered nurse (SRN)	1	infirmière diplômée d'Etat (IDE)
steady (to)	21	stabiliser
stem cell	11	cellule souche
step	17	étape / pas
sterile field	23	champ stérile
sternum	6	sternum
stethoscope	12	stéthoscope
stethoscope bell	19	pavillon de stéthoscope
stethoscope diaphragm	19	membrane de stéthoscope
stick (to)	16	se coller
stick in (to)	17	planter
sticky	13	visqueux
still	22	néanmoins / toutefois
still birth (SB)	24	mort-né
sting (to)	9	piquer
stinging	4	sensation de décharge électrique
stinky	18	malodorant / puant
stitch	4	point de suture
stitch cutter	12	coupe-fil
stomach	11	estomac
stool	22	tabouret (de bain)
storage	15	stockage
storey (US)	2	étage
straight away	6	immédiatement
strain	20	souche
strap	18	bande
strength	1	force
stretch (to)	28	se prolonger
strike (to)	19	frapper

stroke	5	attaque (cérébrale)
stroke	18	passage / application
strong	8	fort
struggle (to)	8	lutter / se débattre
student nurse (GB)	1	étudiant infirmier / infirmière
stuff	10	trucs / choses
sturdy	13	robuste
subside (to)	8	s'atténuer
suction	23	aspiration
sudden infant death syndrome (SIDS)	24	mort subite inopinée du nourrisson
suffer from	10	souffrir de
sufferer	17	malade
suffering	10	souffrance
suit (to)	7	convenir
suitcase	7	valise
summon help (to)	3	appeler à l'aide
superbug	20	bactérie multi-résistante (BMR)
superior vena cava	9	veine cave supérieure
supplies	12	fournitures
supplies and distribution	2	fournitures
supply the needs (to)	13	répondre aux besoins
support (to)	4	soutenir
support person	2	accompagnant
supportive care	27	soins de soutien
suppository	25	suppositoire
suppurating	18	purulent
surface area	13	surface / aire
surgeon	23	chirurgien
surgery	8	opération chirurgicale
surgical	18	chirurgical
surgical floor	23	département de chirurgie
surgical ward	2	département de chirurgie
surname	3	nom de famille
surround (to)	23	entourer
survey	15	enquête
survival	9	survie
survival rate	29	taux de survie
suture set	12	boîte à suture
swab	12	compresse / écouvillon
(alcohol) swab	17	tampon (d'alcool)
swallow (to)	13	avaler
swallowing	13	déglutition
sweep out of (to)	13	extraire de
swing (to)	23	balancer / basculer
switch	7	interrupteur
switch (to)	21	changer de
swivel (to)	22	pivoter
swollen	6	enflé / gonflé / boursouflé
syringe	12	seringue
syrup	25	sirop

T

tablet	25	comprimé
tachycardia	19	tachycardie
tail	21	extrémité du lien
tailor (to)	8	adapter
take a blood sample (to)	21	faire une prise de sang
take a deep breath (to)	13	inspirer profondément
take away (to)	16	enlever / transporter
take into account (to)	1	prendre en compte
take up (to)	10	commencer / se mettre à
tape	18	sparadrap
target (to)	20	cibler
task	15	tâche
taut	18	étiré / tendu
teaching hospital	2	centre hospitalier universitaire (CHU)
team	27	équipe
tear	16	déchirure
teeth (one tooth)	8	dents
temperature (T)	24	température
tend to (to)	14	avoir tendance à
tense	27	tendu
terminally-ill patient	27	patient en phase terminale
testicles / testes (sg. testis)	15	testicules
theatre	2	bloc opératoire
theatre nurse (GB)	1	instrumentiste / panseuse
therefore	10	donc / par conséquent
thigh	4	cuisse
thigh bone	6	fémur
thin	9	fin / mince
thoroughly	23	méticuleusement
thought	26	pensée
thoughtfulness	11	prévenance / bienveillance
thread	23	fil
throat	13	gorge
throbbing	5	pulsatile
throughout	29	tout au long de
thumb	4	pouce
tibia	6	tibia
tick (to)	27	cocher
tickly (cough)	25	(toux) irritante / d'irritation
tidal volume	28	volume courant
tightly	13	fermement
time consuming	14	chronophage
tingly	9	qui picote / qui donne des fourmillements
tiny	11	minuscule
tip	4	bout / extrémité
tired	27	fatigué
toe	4	orteil
toiletries	7	articles de toilette
tongue	8	langue
toothpaste	7	dentifrice
tough	30	dur / difficile
tourniquet	21	garrot

towel	7	serviette
trachea	13	trachée
tracheotomy / tracheostomy (trach)	28	trachéotomie / trachéostomie
train (to)	19	former
training	30	formation
training period	1	stage
trapped	10	coincé / comprimé
tray	12	plateau
treat (to)	11	traiter / soigner
treatment	10	traitement
triage nurse	3	infirmière au triage
trolley (GB)	23	chariot
troopers	30	soldats
trouble	10	ennuis / problèmes
trudge (to)	30	marcher péniblement / patauger
truly	11	véritablement
trust hospital (GB)	30	hôpital
tub	22	baignoire
tubing	16	tubulure
tug (to)	7	tirer (fort)
turn left (to)	2	tourner à gauche
turn on (to)	15	se mettre en marche
turn right (to)	2	tourner à droite
tweezers	12	pince à épiler
twice	9	deux fois
twin	26	jumeau
twin-size day bed	7	canapé d'appoint deux places
twist (to)	6	tordre
tympanic thermometer	12	thermomètre auriculaire
type O blood	21	sang de groupe O

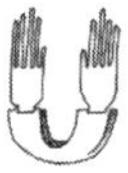

ulna	6	cubitus
unavoidable	12	inévitable
unbearable	5	insupportable
unblock (to)	25	dégager / déboucher
uncertainties	30	aléas
undergo (to)	17	subir
underlying	24	sous-jacent
undernutrition	22	sous-alimentation
understanding	14	compréhensif
undertake (to)	30	entreprendre
underwear	9	sous-vêtements
undress (to)	3	déshabiller
unit	28	unité / service
unless	28	à moins que
unroll (to)	16	dérouler
unsheathe (to)	21	retirer de sa protection
unstick (to)	18	décoller
unwanted	29	indésirable
unwell	28	souffrant / qui ne se sent pas bien
up to	10	jusqu'à
up to date	3	à jour

upper	22	supérieur
upper airways	13	voies respiratoires supérieures
upper jaw	6	mâchoire supérieure
upper limb	4	membre supérieur
upside down	17	à l'envers
upward	14	vers le haut
ureter	15	uretère
urethra	15	urètre
urge	15	besoin pressant / impérieux
urge (to)	11	exhorter / conseiller vivement
urine bottle	15	pistolet
urinary catheter	15	sonde urinaire
urinary tract infection (UTI)	15	infection urinaire
uterine tube	15	trompe de Fallope
uterus / womb	15	utérus

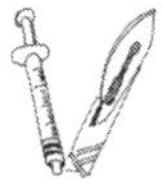

vagina	15	vagin
valuables	28	objets de valeur
valvular heart disease	19	valvulopathie / cardiopathie valvulaire
varicella zoner virus (VZV)	24	virus varicelle-zona
vein	16	veine
venous blood	16	sang veineux
ventilator	23	respirateur / ventilateur
ventricle	9	ventricule
ventricular fibrillation	19	fibrillation ventriculaire
vertebra (pl. vertebrae)	6	vertèbre (vertèbres)
vessel (blood)	16	vaisseau (sanguin)
via	30	par l'intermédiaire de
vial	17	ampoule / fiole
villi (sg. villus)	14	villosités
visiting nurse (US)	1	infirmière à domicile / infirmière libérale
vital signs	3	signes vitaux / constantes

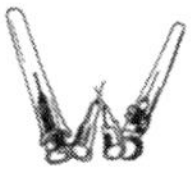

waist	4	taille
waiting room	22	salle d'attente
walking frame	22	déambulateur
wall	13	paroi
ward	1	unité de soins
wardrobe	7	armoire
warm	20	chaud
warn (to)	20	avertir
warning	9	avertissement
washbasin	7	lavabo

washcloth	7	gant de toilette
waste	12	déchet
waste (to)	12	gaspiller
waterborne infection	20	infection d'origine hydrique
waterproof pad	18	champ de soins stérile / imperméable
wave	14	onde
wave (to)	13	osciller
weak	22	faible
weaken (to)	10	affaiblir
weapon	20	arme
wear out (to)	16	s'épuiser
weather	30	temps
weigh (to)	19	peser
weight (Wt)	6	poids
well-being	1	bien-être
wet (to)	20	mouiller
whatever	27	quel que soit
wheelchair	3	fauteuil roulant
wheezing	24	sifflement
whether	27	si
whether ... or	29	que … ou que
(a little) while	28	(un petit) moment
white blood cell (WBC)	16	globule blanc
whole (blood)	16	(sang) entier
wide range of fields	1	large éventail de domaines
widely	22	largement
widowed	3	veuf / veuve
wig	26	perruque
willing	21	consentant
windpipe	13	trachée
wipe	12	lingette
wipe (to)	15	essuyer / désinfecter / nettoyer
wish (to)	26	souhaiter / désirer
with regard to	17	en ce qui concerne
withdraw (to)	21	retirer
withdrawal	26	repli sur soi
wonderful	22	merveilleux / formidablement bien
work wonders (to)	10	faire des merveilles
worry (to)	9	s'inquiéter
wound	4	plaie
wound assessment	30	évaluation des plaies
wound care	30	soins des plaies
wound healing	18	cicatrisation
wrap (to)	19	enrouler
wrinkles	8	rides
wrist	4	poignet
writhe in agony (to)	8	se tordre de douleur
wrong	25	mauvais

X-ray	2	radiologie
X-ray (to)	6	faire une radio

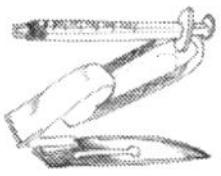

zygomatic bone	6	os zygomatique
Zimmer frame	22	déambulateur

Des mêmes auteurs chez le même éditeur

L'anglais médical à la faculté, Carnet D, Foucher G, Walker P, Jeannin L, 1994.

Words : Sciences de la Santé, Carnet D, Foucher G, Walker P, Jeannin L, 2000.

L'anglais pour la santé – Exercices d'appropriation de la langue à visée professionnelle, Carnet D, Morgan S, Pastore F, 2001.

La communication orale scientifique en anglais. Guide pratique à l'usage des Sciences de la Vie et de la Santé, Carnet D, Charpy JP, Creuzot-Garcher C, 2002.

Préparer son séjour d'étude ou de recherche en pays Anglophone, Carnet D, Charpy JP, Pastore F, Steinmetz E, 2004.

Lexique des termes médicaux, Carnet D, 2006.

L'anglais médical à la faculté, nouvelle édition, Carnet D, Charpy JP, de la Grange P, Bastable P, 2008.

L'anglais pour la santé – Exercices d'appropriation de la langue à visée professionnelle, nouvelle édition, Carnet D, Morgan S, Pastore F, 2008.

L'article de recherche scientifique en anglais, Carnet D, Charpy JP, Bastable P, 2010.

Lexique anglais/français à l'usage des professions paramédicales, Carnet D, 2010.